von Fr. Ulmer

Dipl.-Ing. Torsten K. Keppner
Epfenbergstraße 2-4
74937 Spechbach

D1746585

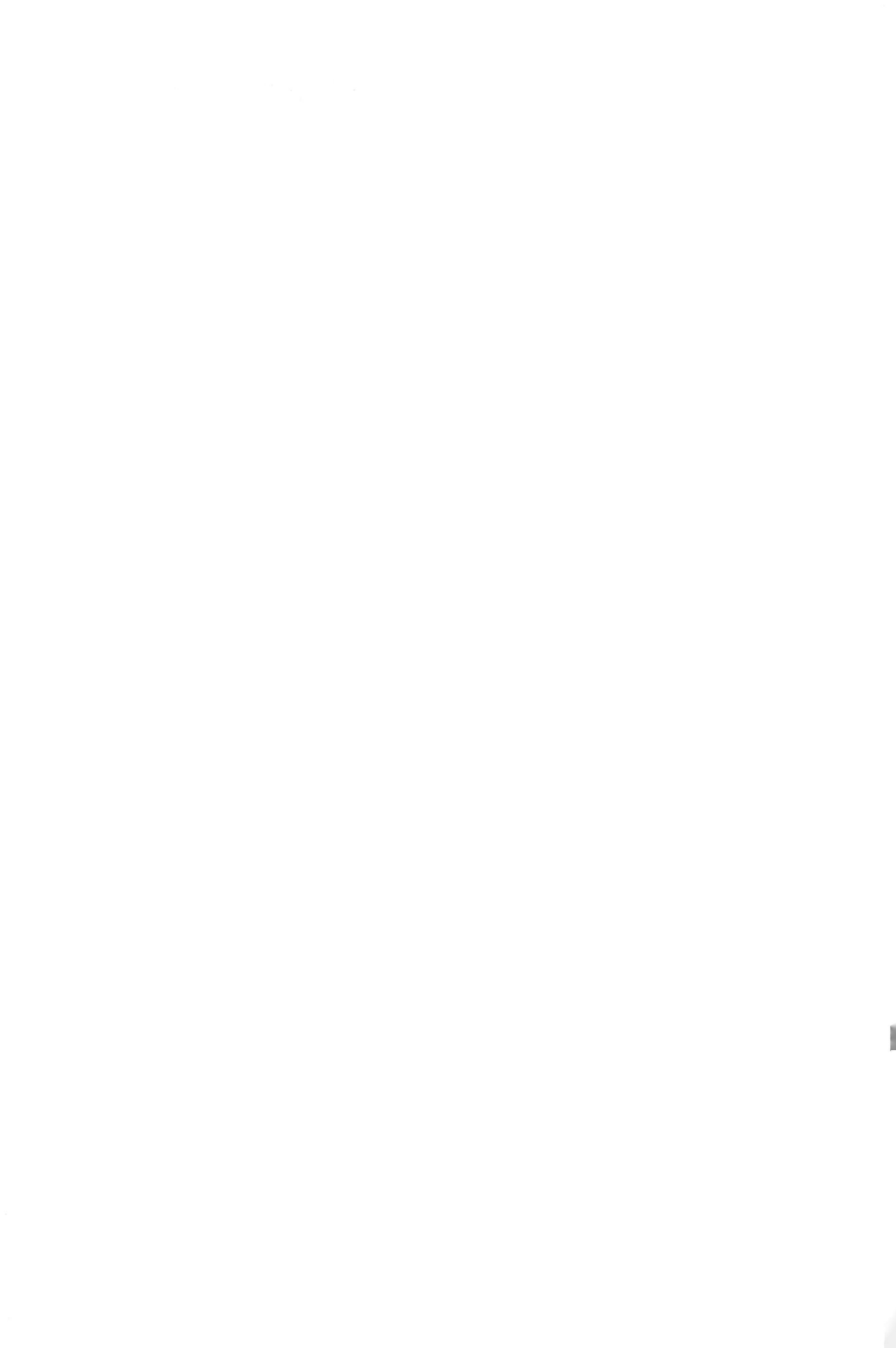

GERONTECHNOLOGY

Why and How

Thomas L. Harrington
Marcia K. Harrington

Produced by

Herman Bouma Foundation for Gerontechnology
http://www.gerontechnology.nl
Eindhoven, the Netherlands

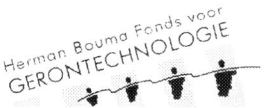

Cover design by:
    Theo M.J. Raijmakers

Produced by:
    Herman Bouma Foundation for Gerontechnology
    http://www.gerontechnology.nl

Copyright Shaker 2000

All rights reserved. No part of this book may be reproduced, stored in a retrieval system, or transmitted, in any form or by any means, without written permission from the publisher.

ISBN 90-423-0107-4
Shaker Publishing B.V.
St. Maartenslaans 26
NL-6221 AX Maastricht
The Netherlands
Phone: + 31 43 350 0424
Fax: + 31 43 325 5090
http://www.shaker.nl

Table of contents

Preface   1

Chapter 1   **Overview of the field**   7
    H. Bouma, J.L. Fozard,
    T.L. Harrington and W.G. Koster

Chapter 2   **Healthy aging**   37
    T.L. Harrington and C.A. Vermeulen

Chapter 3   **Housing**   59
    T.L. Harrington, W.J.M. Heys,
    W.G. Koster and J. Westra

Chapter 4   **Lifelong working**   85
    T.L. Harrington and C.A. Vermeulen

Chapter 5   **Personal Mobility and Transportation**   115
    T.L. Harrington, J. Rietsema and
    M. Vercruyssen

Chapter 6   **Information and Communication**   139
    H. Bouma and T.L. Harrington

Chapter 7   **Mathematical modeling and simulation**   165
    P. Bidyuk, J.A.M. Graafmans,
    T.L. Harrington and M.L.J. Hautus

Chapter 8   **Gerontechnology unfolding**   187
    H. Bouma, D.G. Bouwhuis and
    J.E.M.H. van Bronswijk

Bibliography	**207**
Keyword index	**217**
Author index	**221**
Index boxes	**223**
Index figures	**225**

Preface

Imagine yourself when you are 60 years old, or 80. What will your life and your activities be like? Will you do new, exciting things or the same things you like to do now? Will you be able to do simple things such as reading the paper, taking a bath, turning on the stereo, driving a car or taking money from a cash-dispenser? Where will you live, and in what kind of house? Will you be able to enjoy new freedom from a life of work and develop new ambitions? Will you be independent?

When asked, older people say that continuing to maintain independence as they grow older is very important to them. Indeed, independence is a quality of adult life in our society that we cherish at any age. Being able to live independently and being able to do what you want partly depends on your health and abilities, but also on the relevant social and physical environment. A supportive environment can help people continue doing what they are accustomed to and doing new things they want to do, even though they may perhaps see or hear somewhat less well, move with more difficulty, or have somewhat poorer memories.

The social part of a supportive environment is composed of people (family, friends, or if needed professional caregivers) who provide help.
The physical part includes technology that makes living easier and more enjoyable.

Throughout life, technology helps persons with products (hardware, software, and services), which provide a large range of possibilities in perception, communication, information processing, and mobility, and in maintaining health. Technology can meet daily needs when it is useful, easy to use, and available at a reasonable cost.

What is gerontechnology?

The term gerontechnology is a composite of two words, "gerontology," the scientific study of aging and "technology": research, development and design of new and improved techniques, products, and services. Gerontology is concerned with research on the biological, psychological, social, and medical aspects of aging. Technology includes all branches of relevant scientific endeavor: physical, chemical, civil, mechanical, electrical, industrial, information, and communication engineering.

Gerontechnology refers to technology that fulfills the need of an aging society, i.e. research, development, and design in the engineering disciplines based on scientific knowledge about the aging process. So it is technology in direct contact with insights into ambitions and needs of aging people in their environment and the aging process itself. More formally, gerontechnology is defined as the study of technology and aging for ensuring good health, full social participation, and independent living throughout the entire life span, however much it may lengthen.

Five roads are to be paved to address the technological challenges of aging in society both for men and women:

First, technology can be used effectively in prevention of age-related diseases and of age-associated losses in strength, endurance, and other physical or cognitive abilities. Technology can play an important role in primary prevention of potential losses and in secondary prevention of unwanted consequences of existing disease or loss. Research has shown that these losses are modifiable through interventions such as improved nutrition, physical exercise, a healthier environment, and modifications of life style. The preventive role of technology includes the design of equipment to facilitate interventions and the design of monitoring equipment that allows feedback about compliance with interventions and their effectiveness. Examples include strength training equipment that is stimulating to use or safety equipment for persons using dangerous tools.

Second, gerontechnology can enhance the performance and opportunities of older citizens in new roles that fit their new ambitions. The new roles include changed work, leisure, living, and modified social situations.

The potential for technology in these areas has not been developed to a significant degree up to now. An example is the development of user-friendly communication technology to facilitate remote contacts, to make new contacts and to participate in educational activities. The emphasis here is on what older people want to do and can do, rather than on what they cannot, such as running the 100 meter in 10 seconds.

Third, it provides technology to compensate for declining capacities, the challenge of aging. This is the most fully developed aspect of gerontechnology and includes products and techniques to compensate for physical, perceptual, and cognitive losses, and for task redesign that takes into account, for example, longer response times. An example here is reading glasses to compensate for diminishing flexibility of the eye's lens.

Fourth, gerontechnology provides technical support that assists caregivers who care for less able older persons. Take for example technology for lifting and transferring persons who are incapable of moving themselves. Many products have been developed for use in hospitals and rehabilitation facilities and some of this technology is currently or potentially available.

Fifth, technology aids older persons indirectly by improving research on aging. In many studies on aging, the technological environment and the technological options are not yet taken into account. For example, technology allows imaging organs and tissues, signal processing of neurological events and making other non-invasive measurements, thereby revolutionizing the scientific study of the processes within the aging body.

Some central ideas

Three concepts are central to gerontechnology:

The first concept is that the dynamics of society is driven by technological developments, in particular related to information and communication technology. If older people are to remain integrated into society, technology should explicitly be directed to the fast growing segment of independent older citizens.

The second is that age-associated differences in ambitions and in functioning of men and women can be met by improvements in the technological environment. Suitable information and communication tools can for example serve an ambition. A task that may seem very difficult to an older person in one situation may be easily accomplished with suitable environmental modifications. The very idea of age grading of ambitions and of abilities cannot be considered independently of the technological environment.

The third concept is that older citizens should remain in control of their technological environment i.e. they should be enabled to decide what they want to be done automatically or by robots. This refers to the concept of the user interface between older users and useful technology.

About this book

This is the first textbook in gerontechnology. In recent years there has been an explosion of interest and involvement in this new field.
Yet there has been no basic text for use in formal and informal education. Specialists in basic and applied technology who might wish to contribute to the quality of life of older people, and gerontologists who see a need to channel more technology to older persons might also benefit from a basic text. And there are potential participants among the general public: the curious, the concerned, those with older friends or relatives, people growing older, which includes us all, and the aged themselves.

Our plan for dealing with this complex task was simple. Gerontechnology reaches into every vein of technology, but no one author can know every domain. So we decided to entrain a group of experts for each of the various chapters. We had lengthy discussions and seminars with the experts and with interested older people, who also are experts. So in an interactive process between the editors and the experts, the chapters took shape.

Next, because the book could never cover the full scope of gerontechnology, we decided on a few exemplar fields of technology that we could use in the book to epitomize the problems, solutions, cautions, hopes, and dreams of gerontechnology. Accordingly, we focused individual chapters on the relation of older people to the technologies of five principle areas. These were longevity and health, housing, working, mobility and transportation, and informational systems and communication. In addition to these, to exemplify the involvement of the sciences and tie everything together, we included mathematical modeling and simulation. The book begins and ends with general chapters on gerontechnology.

The book evolved at the former Institute for Gerontechnology of Eindhoven University of Technology, and was later taken over by the Herman Bouma Foundation for Gerontechnology. Fruitful connections were made with the more recent thematic network GENIE: Gerontechnology Education Network In Europe, in which over 40 European universities collaborate to develop and harmonize their curriculum in Gerontechnology. The GENIE thematic network is funded by the European Commission and will be continued as a standing committee of the International Society for Gerontechnology.

Acknowledgements

A host of informal contributors provided a mountain of technical substance in our discussions, meetings and seminars. Apart from the authors of the chapters, they are in alphabetical order:

Ad van Berlo, Ph.D., Chris de Bruijn, Ph.D., Mili Docampo Rama, M.Sc., Leslie Harrington, M.D., Ralph Herbig, M.A., D.O., Fred Huf, Ph.D., Maddy Janse, Ph.D., Jan Kok, Ph.D., Wiet Koren, Ph.D., Teddy McCalley, Ph.D., Curt Mearns, Ph.D., Marilyn Melton, Ko Rijpkema, Ph.D., Yvonne Slangen-de Kort, Ph.D., Mariëlle Snijders, M.Sc., Robert Solso, Ph.D., Windy de Weerd, M.Sc..

We are grateful to all of them.

Herman Bouma Foundation for Gerontechnology
http://www.gerontechnology.nl

CHAPTER ONE

Overview of the Field

Gerontechnology, as its name suggests, is an interdiscipline that discovers and deploys technology on behalf of people in their maturing years. Its domain includes gerontology, the study of aging, together with the wide spectrum of technologies that come from engineering, mathematics, and from physical and biological sciences.

In gerontechnology, we assess the circumstances of older individuals and their own attitudes toward them, recursively modeling, theorizing, designing, testing, then re-assessing and re-designing. We ask people in the range over fifty or sixty what is missing from their lives and then search through the technical artifacts, modern and ancient, looking for tools that will be useful to people as they age. The candidates range from computer systems to recreational devices to new kinds of spectacles. If some promising tool doesn't fit hands or minds, it is reshaped. If a new tool is too complicated, too unfamiliar, too sharp or too dull or otherwise unsatisfactory, then the gerontechnologist tries to reformulate the tool or recruits some specialists to forge it into a supportive and useable form.

Gerontechnology's importance is increasing because of the growing number of individuals experiencing the decades from 50 onwards, even up through 100 or more. We have elected to call these the maturing years, a period of fruition, gradual bodily changes and commensurate mental and physical adaptations. The maturing years are a period of ongoing contribution and productivity as well as a period of reaping rewards from earlier effort. World wide, the numerical increase in those getting to enjoy this rich period in the life span is swelling for several reasons. Their number is increasing partly because the general population is increasing and partly because people are living longer and longer with improved diet, medical care and public health measures. They are increasingly prominent in society as the birth rate also drops.

The number of people living independently as opposed to being in institutional care, shown as a function of age and gender can be seen in Figure 1.1, emphasizing how much we need to change some of our stereotypes about life in the maturing period.

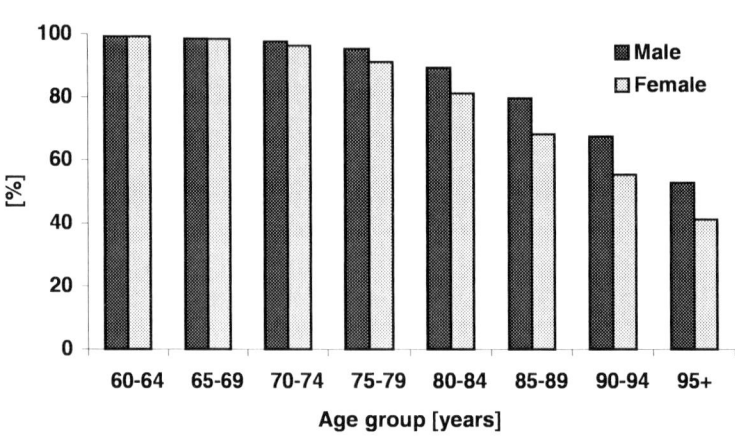

Figure 1.1 Percentage of people living independently in the Netherlands (as of January 1996). Data from Statistics Netherlands/Statline.

The figure makes clear that the majority of older people are living independently. Only some 8 percent of the population over 60 years is living in an institution. All others are living independently with or without external help. It is predicted that the percentage of people living in an institution will further decrease from the actual 8% in 1996 to about 4% in 2020. As a consequence, the request for home care will increase.

One face of technology's leverage: refurbishment

Most people, as they age, really don't change very much from year to year. Nevertheless there are some slow changes that people experience that accumulate and may become somewhat annoying, and there are other changes that perhaps improve the person in some way. One of the tasks of gerontechnology is to facilitate refurbishment of people's individual capabilities. An aging pianist may need new joints in some fingers, an artist may need to have plastic lenses implanted in both eyes, or some of us may require new hips to help us re-enter normal daily life.

On the crest of technology not in the trough

In addition to applying technology on behalf of people, in a sense part of gerontechnology involves saving them from it. Advances in technology change society, and technology never stops changing; it keeps on moving like a tidal wave as human knowledge increases. Thus, at the same time it both causes new problems and offers new solutions. Just as a surfer's momentary inattention and minute deviation while riding on the wave can abruptly and irreparably disrupt the ride, so can falling behind the wave of technology precipitously disrupt a life. Often this means that people who don't keep up will face technical, perhaps social isolation, and will suffer in productivity and gratification. One has to adapt continually to remain a fully participating citizen of the world. So, teaching technology, after reformatting it so that it is easily understood by people who grew up in different eras, is part of the task. We must think of new ways to allow older people to train themselves. The establishment of computerized drop-in centers with adequate help on hand is one answer.

Gerontechnology: a positive movement

Although "geron" stems from the Greek for "old man," the field of gerontechnology steadfastly avoids the common stereotypes surrounding "old" because they apply to so few of older people. Most older people are healthy, intelligent, actively energetic, and wise humans. Primarily, it is these vigorous individuals with whom gerontechnology tends to deal, though the minority who do have significant deficits are also included, both because of their deficits and because apart from the deficits they are normal older people.

Box 1.1 Demography of age

How many older people are there?

Average life expectancy has increased worldwide from 48 years in 1955, to 65 years in 1995 and will increase to an expected 73 years in 2025. Although the trend is similar in all countries the absolute values greatly differ between the various regions.

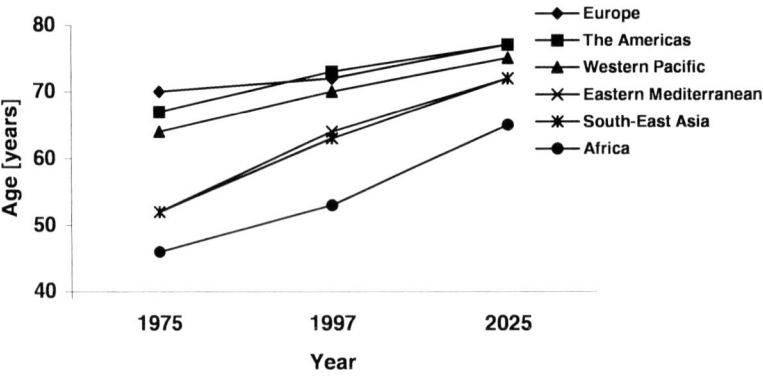

**Figure 1 Life expectancy at birth in various continents.
Based on data from The World Health Report 1998, p.39.**

In the least developed countries (LDC) today 3 out of 4 people are still dying before the age of 50, compared to 2 out of 5 worldwide. Ten million of these deaths are among children under 5 years.

The total fertility rate (TFR) (number of births per woman of childbearing age) declined from 5 in 1955 to 2.9 in 1995. It is expected to reach 2.3 by 2025. In many countries the fertility rate is too low for the population to remain stable. The mean number of children per family in Italy is 1.2 and to have the population remain stable, a mean number of 2.1 is required.
The world average, however, conceals large differences among countries and regions. TFRs in 1995 ranged from 1.2 in Italy to 7.6 in Yemen.
In 1995 the TFR for the developed world was only 1.7 compared with 5.4 for the LDCs.

As a consequence of the increasing contraceptive measures worldwide the values are converging.

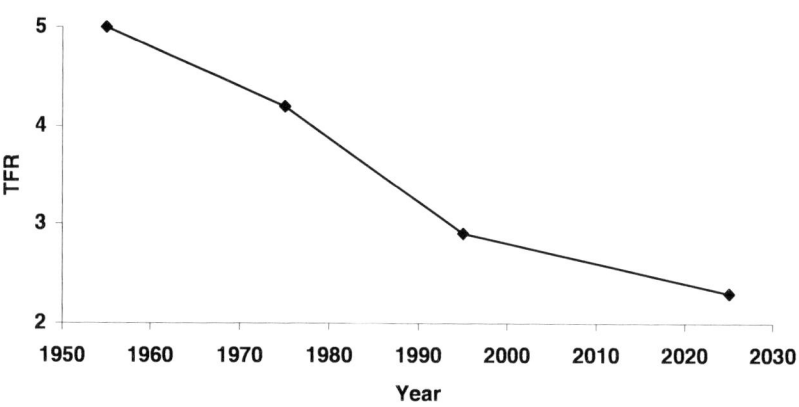

Figure 2 Decrease in total fertility rate over the years worldwide. Data from The World Health Report 1998, p. 119-120.

Due to these trends the world population is still growing from 5.8 billion in 1997 to an expected 8 billion in 2025. In the developed countries the fertility rates are low, life expectancy is high and population will remain stabile. The consequence is that the mean age of the population in the developed countries will increase. Already in 1994 Italy had reached the point where the older people (60+) outnumbered the children under 16. France will reach this point in 2009 and the USA in 2027. Back in the fifties Italy had 3 times more young people than older people.
The process of an aging population will continue into the next decades.

This aging population will have a major impact on the social and economic structure of the countries and will have political ramifications within each country.

World Health Organization. (1998). The World Health Report. Life in the 21st century: a vision for all. World Health Organization, Geneva. ISBN 92-4-156189-0.

Throughout this book we encourage you in similar fashion to focus your thinking toward the positive. Consider some of the more glamorous sides of aging, for instance, freedom to travel and to indulge in recreation. One's views of this field are largely colored by whether we see ourselves as helping older people to "hold the line" against the passage of time, or by whether we see something more fundamental and exciting still: the possibility of a stage in life when humans for the first time in history have the possibility of combining leisure time and reasonable health for continued creativity and productivity, and perhaps using their spirit and energy for human advancement in ways we cannot presently conceive.

Inspiration from a history of fortuitous successes

Even though most older people are fit, some things still may change with age as indicated above. We may see our reaction times getting somewhat longer and may notice overall strength becoming somewhat less. Then our thoughts turn to prosthetics. A substantial proportion of the population is in bifocals by age 50.

Presently, there are many striking victories in gerontechnology against such changes. On the medical front, beta blockers, diuretics, and pacemakers artificially regulate the basic essentials such as blood pressure, fluid levels, and cardiac rhythms, allowing people who might otherwise be incapacitated to perform normally. Improving on one of the greatest aids of all time, eyeglasses, varifocal glasses have been developed to give continuous gradations of optical correction, avoiding the bifocal "line" and the regions of misfocus that bifocals cause. There are countless mechanical devices that benefit aging people, which allow the very weak to build strength gradually. With one such device the user stands on a small platform and performs pull-ups with the arms. The hydraulic platform offsets some of the strength required. Lighting standards have been raised on behalf of older people, and there are even buses that bend their knees, like camels, so that the more frail older people don't have to bend their own knees so much when boarding.
Now, inspired by the past successes, the formal field of gerontechnology is being evolved as a deliberate and organized movement designed specifically to engineer the breakthroughs that will let people not only hold the line, but often become better than they were before as they explore their new horizons.

Our primary goal in this book

Throughout the ensuing chapters we will delineate the field of gerontechnology as it applies to specific issues and areas, and we will point out opportunities for you the reader to become personally involved. At the very least, we hope to interest you in parts of the field by illustrating some of the special applications of the gerontechnology movement. How do we define and delimit the territory? What is our vantage point over the vast terrain of aging and the aged? What means are available to us for helping the aged and how should we search for others? Is there some niche you yourself might enjoy filling? Obviously, the field is interdisciplinary to the extreme. Just about anyone from any field can offer major contributions. The gerontechnologist may be a specialist, say a chemist or an inventor, or may be a generalist or just a person who is interested and likes to think and act. Nearly every technologist is a potential gerontechnologist. And nearly every scientist too has a place in the field, performing scientific experiments to arrive at new insights, developing technology, inventing, foraging, forging, educating or politicizing.

The spirit of the book

Gerontechnology lives primarily in the future. Certainly there are countless instances in the past where technology was applied to some problem of older people. But past solutions aren't the province of the field of gerontechnology because solutions that are achieved are relegated to fields such as recreation, health care or gerontology or medicine once they have been developed and implemented. Rather, this field focuses on problems that have yet to be solved, and even more murky, on problems that have yet to be discovered. For this reason, we won't adopt the goal of books in many fields, of transferring large bodies of information about the field's specific problems and answers from the past to readers' memories.
We concur with Albert Einstein's statement that imagination is more important than (memorizing) knowledge.

Still, a framework of solid knowledge often helps. There are many roads to the solution of any gerontechnological problem. In order to improve on eyeglasses you might profit by bringing along some knowledge of the physiological optics of the human eye, and some physical optics of lenses. Or you might know something about the relevant facts of perception, or about neurophysiology. But maybe not. You might approach the problem with totally different information and a different style, perhaps simply proceeding by way of your own experimentation. Your tack is your own choice and will depend on your field and on your previous training and personal style and on the prevailing winds. Nevertheless, we will regularly supply useful relevant knowledge that is at least suggestive of possible solutions and directions for thought by providing examples.

But, instead of solving many concrete examples and practicing with algorithms to obtain solutions as is done in teaching algebra, we hope to challenge the reader with the many unsolved problems that older people face and present general ways of thinking about them. Instead of methodically presenting formulas and facts to be memorized we may more often just wave enthusiastically at some general amorphous panorama of concerns for older people, and gesture, as enthusiastically if somewhat vaguely, toward sources of technological power that might be applicable. The intent in doing this is to show the reader where the piles of questions are and where the piles may be, where answers might be found, and then encourage the reader to be the one to carve out and deal with the specifics–find a problem, discover some technology that will work, put them together, maybe define a new problem, devise a better bicycle or design a healthy building, improve an interface or make some machine, write about it, motivate a politician, interest a business man, develop a market, get some funding, perhaps start a new movement. If, from reading this book, the reader takes personal license to try any of these activities, whether the reader's success is mountainous or modest, we will feel that we have succeeded.

The ambitions of older people

The identification of the desires and ambitions of older people is our first task. Second, we must identify opportunities for satisfying them. In this a modified golden rule of technology applies: Try to put the aged in the position that you would like to be put in yourself–but allow for individual differences. On the one hand, older people of course have the obvious basic desires shared by us all. People want to be safe from accidents, hunger, medical problems, animals, and crime, and they want to feel safe from all of these and feel good about the world and about themselves. They want access to other people, to transportation to the bank and the store, to places

Box 1.2 Technophobia?

Many older users make less use of certain recent technologies. Does it follow that they are afraid of using technology? They use electric light, telephone, TV, and public transport normally. So they are not afraid of technology as such. Why might they refrain from using recent information and communication technology? We offer the following suggestions:

Older people may not think the functions offered worth the price. For example, ads about personal computers give technical details, rather than useful functions. A brand of processor is not the same as a useful function.

Older users may not think the assumed functions worth the assumed effort of learning to use the device. User interfaces are generally complex and not at all designed for perceptual, cognitive, and motor functions of older people. Directions of use may be unusable if not lost, and help functions are notorious for being unhelpful (Stewart, 1992).

Older people may have got used to a different type of control as required by menu navigation. They may have learned earlier in life that a device must be treated with proper care and that unbounded exploration by trial-and-error may cause disruption of the device or even danger. People can learn up till any huge age, but unlearning is far more difficult than learning.

Older people may have experienced embarrassment or insecurity when attempting to use a money teller or ticket automat with a queue of people pressing from behind and the apparatus not geared to a slower or inexperienced use.

So, there are many valid reasons from the point of view of older people to be somewhat restrictive in buying and trying to use new information and communication technology. For useful applications, however, the gap must be bridged between older people and the information society that they live in (Lawton, 1998). Otherwise they may fall behind in being fully participating members of their own society. The task of technology and of business is to increase transparency and usability of ICT to the extent that older people can easily learn and like to use it (Bouma, 2000).

Bouma, H. (2000). Document and user interface design for older citizens. In: P.H. Westendorp, C.J.M. Jansen & R. Punselie. (Eds.). Interface Design and Document Design. Rodopi Press, Amsterdam/Atlanta. ISBN 90-420-0510-6.

Lawton, M.P. (1998) Future Society and Technology. In: J.Graafmans, V.Taipale & N.Charness. (Eds). Gerontechnology: A sustainable investment in the future (pp.12-22). IOS Press, Amsterdam. ISBN 90-5199-367-6.

Stewart, T. (1992). Physical interfaces or "obviously it's for the elderly, it's grey, boring and dull." In: H. Bouma & J.A.M. Graafmans (Eds.). Gerontechnology. Proceedings of the first International Conference on Gerontechnology, Eindhoven, August 1991. (pp. 197-207). IOS Press, Amsterdam. ISBN 90-5199-072-3.

across town and perhaps across the continents and oceans. They want freedom from cleaning the oven and from other aggravating work but conversely they need to be able to exercise their human capacities for doing things and solving problems, creating things and accomplishing goals: all people need successes, lots of them. But sometimes technology spells personal failure when one feels unable to keep pace with new technologies as others do.

Each person is unique, and his or her individual situation may make him or her even more so. Also, although many of the things that any given person wants may stay the same, options for obtaining these things may change, again, on a highly individualistic basis that depends on age, socio-economic, political and other factors. All of these must be incorporated into our assessments of desire.

Diversity of the target group

Just as there is diversity in individual desires, older people are scattered widely along most other physical, physiological, and psychological dimensions of description. Older people will have more divergent life histories and environments and abilities than younger people do. Also, there are gender differences that must be considered, which are increasing in importance. Ordinarily, in designing assistance for special groups the case can be rather simple: put in ramps for the people in wheel chairs, give the people who have trouble with locomotion special parking places, and so on. But most older people don't belong neatly to such groups. They aren't even close to being in wheel chairs, and they don't have trouble with locomotion. So there is an evident need for caution against stereotyping. The answer of course is flexible action that is sensitive to what the older people seem to want and what they don't want. But this target can be very counterintuitive. Signs in parking places are beginning to spring up, "For persons over 65," nice for those who need them, but most seniors can probably be expected to drive disdainfully past, leaving them for people who are really old. Older people don't usually think of themselves as being old. These people may appreciate other kinds of assistance more, such as the free passes that some ski areas are offering to those over seventy.

The solutions for good design proposed here all stress this same flexibility and individuality of solutions, geared to the individual, not the average. An example is the rheostat-controlled dimmer that allows an individual to set the intensity level of the light so that viewing various things by a wide assortment of visual systems is easy and comfortable.

Golden rule number two: Give unto others...

The original golden rule, "Do unto others as you would have them do unto you," requires another minor modification here. Give unto others things they want to have, not things we want to give. Gerontechnology is in part a "helping" movement. It is human nature to want to give as much as possible when trying to help someone. So there is the common danger of giving too much, giving things that aren't wanted, or things that will be unpleasant or turn out to be even harmful. In gerontechnology our large arsenal of ideas and devices and methods especially predisposes us to this, the "bear's favor", a Russian expression for favors gone wrong. In some countries good Samaritans are even legally responsible for the ill effects of bad favors.

To avoid the bear's favor, we have to determine carefully and exactly what is needed, but therein lies yet another problem. People often don't know what they actually want because all of the options and their advantages and consequences aren't obvious. Here the marketing facet of gerontechnology comes into play in advertising the kinds of opportunities that are available. The technology of market research can be used to determine what people prefer. It can also be used to assess satisfaction of older users.

Box 1.3 Change in sex ratio

In the older segments of the population (65+) women typically outnumber men. This is a worldwide phenomenon that is observed in nearly all countries. A rare exception is India. Worldwide the sex ratio, i.e. the number of female per male, is 1.32, whereas in India the ratio is 0.99. On the other hand is the sex ratio extremely high in Russia, where at the age of 65 years and higher on each male are 2.27 females.

The situation in the United States is rather characteristic for the situation elsewhere in the Western world.
In 1950 the sex ratio of women to men 65 years and older in the United States was 1.12. In 1990 the sex ratio had increased to 1.49, and of all women in the United States in 1990, 14.7% were older than 65, whereas only 10.4% of the men were over 65, as indicated in the inset.

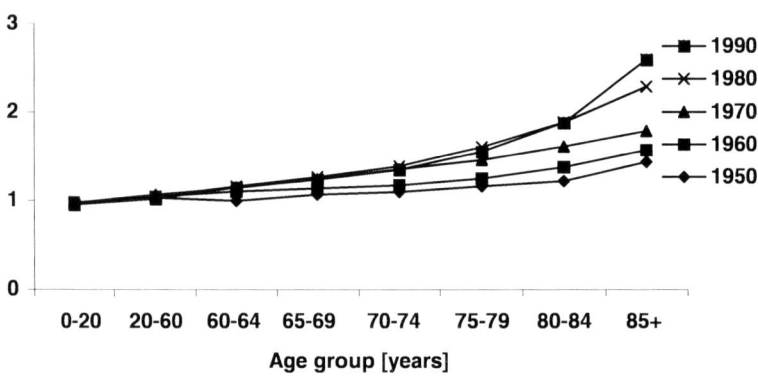

Figure 1 Ratios of females to males in the United States in different age groups and in various years. Data from US Census Bureau
(http://www.census.gov/ipc/www/idbsprd.html).

As can be observed in Figure 1 the preponderance of women over men is growing with age. The sex ratio for those over 80 was in 1990 2.59, which means that about 70% of the 80+ people were women.
As you would expect, the relative difference between numbers of men and women is greatest among the centenarians, people over 100.

For instance of all centenarians in the Netherlands in 1997 83% were women, which implies a sex ratio of 4.88. The total number of centenarians in the Netherlands increased over the past years from 165 in 1970 to 1006 in 1997. The number of centenarians among men increased from 60 in 1970 to 218 in 1990 and then decreased to 171 and among women it increased from 105 in 1970 to 835 in 1997 (Brekel, 1998).

It is predicted that the preponderance of women over men will increase in the coming years. For the United States from 2020 on a gradual decrease is predicted as can be seen in Figure 2.

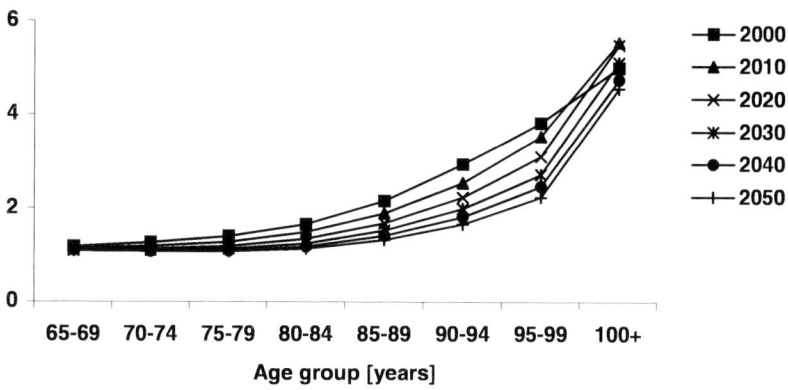

Figure 2 Predicted ratios of females to males in the United States in various age groups and its changes over the years. Data from U.S. Census Bureau
(http://www.census.gov/population/projections/nation/nas/npas.txt).

The existence of an older population that is predominantly female has important implications for gerontechnology. The balance of planning and allocation should shift toward the particular characteristics of older women, whose needs and vulnerabilities are different from those of older men.

Brekel, H. van den. (1998). Demos, 14(2), 4p.
http://www.nidi.nl/public/demos/dm98024.html

U.S. Consensus Bureau http://www.census.gov

Getting involved in gerontechnology

You, the reader, may want to get started immediately, working on some problem in gerontechnology. Suppose you are concerned with the sensory motor performance of older people. A viable course of action might go something like the following.

First, you need to formulate the problem of interest. It is nearly always informative to get opinions and suggestions from some of older people themselves to be sure that your perception of the problem is realistic. Next, you may find it useful to survey the literature of any branches of science and technology that could apply, and to interview specialists, if required, to accumulate the pertinent facts and theories.

Armed with this information, you can gain further insight into many problems of sensory motor performance by simulating them. You put yourself in the position of older people. To get a feel for this, you might try a quick "pilot study." Try telephoning wearing 30 dB earplugs or even with pieces of paper or wet cotton in your ears. Try reading some warning signs, or the label of an over the counter medicine through two or three pairs of sunglasses. Make some appropriate measurements, such as how far away you can read the labels with and without the glasses. Then if the informal results are of interest, you become more formal.
Use neutral density filters instead of sunglasses, and use more standard stimuli, such as an eye chart. Go back to the literature on aging hearing or vision to ensure that your simulation is valid, is representative of what older people would experience. Next, your results can be analyzed and modeled and a theory developed and tested in adherence with the scientific method: hypothesize, test, refine, etc. This theory is simply your conception, based on your information and experiments, of what the circumstances are for older people. This new information can be reformulated as a design standard, or you may simply want to have a demonstration to show to designers or students. Possibly you will want to develop and manufacture and distribute a "fix" for the problem.

As an example on the motor side of human activity, suppose that you were interested in the effects of tremor on motor performance. First, you would determine whether tremor is really a problem, and find out how tremor manifests itself, perhaps by interviewing some older people. If something doesn't cause specific problems of course there is no reason for "fixes."

You would then visit the medical literature to learn what types of tremor, normal and abnormal, have been discovered. There you would also learn their amplitudes and frequencies and find out the circumstances of occurrence, whether they occur during motion, or only during inactivity. Then you would be in a position to simulate some of these tremors using an appropriate vibrator attached to the arm as the individual performed tasks such as spooning liquid, turning pages, positioning a mouse, writing, and so on to determine the extent to which there were debilitating effects on the performance of different tasks and to characterize them. You might then test some people with real tremor to validate your findings, to see if their natural tremors hampered them more or less to the same degree. At this point you would have a type of "age simulator." Next, a mathematical model of the task and of the tremor could be devised that would allow you to predict performance, given a specific amount and type of tremor and given a specific task. Finally, you might choose to develop some "fixes." You could experiment with loading the hand, or with other devices, again measuring performance–pages turned per second perhaps. Having completed your experimentation or at least some observations, you might again think of developing a marketable product. Or you might comb the environment of older people looking for instances of tasks that become difficult because of tremor. Finally, you might want to write an article to alert other people to the problem.

In general, depending on your application, your experimentation may either be of the "shade tree" variety, quick and dirty but adequate for producing the information you need, or you may run thousands of trials that adhere rigidly to the precepts and cautions of standard psychophysics. That is, you might simply view some dimly lit stair or walkway that you fear might cause trouble for older people through glasses that you had smoked with a match to dim your own vision, or you could take the problem into a vision laboratory.

If no problem comes to your mind that you would like to investigate, of course a problem can usually be generated by first considering solutions that exist and "thinking backward"–noticing powerful methods in science and engineering and then looking for applications for them among older people. Examples are e-mail and the Internet.

Box 1.4 Choice reaction time versus typing

A rather common measure of age effects is the measurement of reaction time. As early as 1951 Welford published for the Nuffield Foundation an interim statement under the title "Skill and Age: An experimental Approach." In 1958 the final and updated version was published. In his book a clear distinction is made between organic capacities that decrease with age and experience that increases with age. Depending on the balance between these effects age will either have a positive or negative effect on task performance.
Salthouse (1984) showed the effect of age and skill in typing.

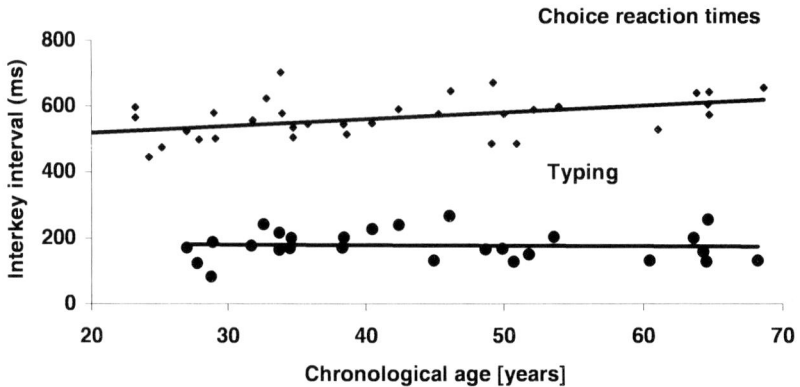

Figure 1 Choice reaction time and typing speed as a function of age. (Data from Salthouse, 1984.)

As the Figure indicates, there is some difference in performance between young and old on this specific task of choice reaction time, a task where the subject doesn't simply respond as quickly as possible to the stimulus, but rather has to make a choice. It appears that the older people take a bit more time to respond. Based on this data one might be inclined to generalize that "You slow down as you get older." However, the data on typing doesn't indicate that older people are slower, per se. The time between keystrokes is about the same for young and old.
Can we still say though that older people are slower on some tasks?
Not yet. For instance, notice that the slowest reaction in the entire group is from a person who is only about 33 years old.

Notice that two fifty-year-olds are quicker than all but two of the entire population is.

Furthermore, we sometimes tend to forget that the data in the graph didn't come from the same persons as they aged, but from a large group of different people of different ages. Perhaps there are a few people in the older group that are slowed, or a few people in the younger group that are faster, perhaps there are some athletes from a college population.

We have to ask not only who is slower but also why they are slow. Among the older population in general there will be more people with Alzheimer's, perhaps as yet undiagnosed, and other factors that slow one down. The older people also don't accommodate their vision as well, a fact that is very commonly ignored in visual experiments. So the experimental statement from these data might really be saying that people with diseases of the nervous system are slower, or that people in general don't respond to things that they don't see well. Statements such as this have nothing to do with age of individuals, per se, even though it may seem that they do. In assessing the effects of age we have to beware and not be led quickly to conclusions.
Moraal (1993) lists an appropriate set of cautions that we need to follow when we talk about declining capabilities.
Which capabilities do we mean, exactly?
What kinds of tasks call for these capabilities and under what circumstances? What is the amount of loss, and can we measure it? When is the onset of a loss? Are there any other factors besides age that might be responsible for a loss? What do we know about compensating mechanisms that might be offsetting a loss?

Moraal, J. (1993). Aging and work. In: K. Broekhuis, C. Weiers & J. Moraal. (Eds.). Aging and human factors. Proceedings of the Europe chapter of the Human Factors and Ergonomics Society. (pp. 7-18). University of Groningen, Groningen. ISBN 90-6807-311-7.

Salthouse, T.A. (1984). Effects of Age and Skill in Typing. Journal of Experimental Psychology, (113) 3, 345-371.

Welford, A.T. (1951). Skill and Age: An experimental approach.
Published for the Nuffield Foundation by the Oxford University Press, London.

Welford, A.T. (1958). Ageing and Human Skill.
Published for the Nuffield Foundation by the Oxford University Press, London.

Five major aspects of gerontechnology

If you have already begun to organize your thinking about the ways that we can keep the doors of opportunity open for older people you probably have noticed that gerontechnology's assorted remedies and activities seem to fall into categories. For instance, we might classify activities in terms of Observation, Prevention, Assistance, and Repair; or possibly Physical Exercise, Mental Exercise, and Social Exercise.
Of course, there are hundreds of such possible groupings.

Without meaning to endorse one specific jargon over the others, and keeping in mind that such classifications are rather arbitrary and should not be viewed as concrete entities, let us introduce one standard partitioning that is used in the field to help organize thinking and action. For reference here we call this grouping, "The five aspects of gerontechnology."

In order to introduce this terminology, let's imagine older people for whom some of the options for normal living are changing. Suppose for instance that we are concerned with retired people with extra free time, or with the decline of happiness of people who are becoming lonely because of diminished ambulatory mobility–they aren't walking as much or as well as they did previously. When technology is required, its applications can usually be grouped, often loosely and perhaps with some ambiguity, into five aspects.
They are Enhancement, Prevention, Compensation, Care, and Research.

When technology serves to help create an environment in which new ambitions of older age can flourish, we may speak of enhancement. The concept is used in the sense of providing self-fulfillment and enrichment through completely different forms of activity or environmental stimulation. The persons might turn to the technology of communication to fill life with new social outlets using computerized e-mail, the Internet, voice mail, or a videophone. If the persons liked to collect stamps they could instantly be in close contact with thousands of other people who enjoyed stamp collecting. Collecting, of all other sorts, gardening discussions, business or professional opportunities, and vast informational services would be fruits of this enhancing form of gerontechnology.
This new wonderland might well replace the joys of going to the store or to the club a hundred fold.

Prevention, from many points of view, is the most important gift that gerontechnology can offer a society as a whole because of the vast sums of money that can be saved and applied to other societal necessities and luxuries. When the billion dollars related to broken hips in the United States alone is added to the astounding expense of cardiac, metabolic, mental, and other ailments and accidents, which could have been staved off by preventive gerontechnology, its image as a cornucopia of benefits for governments and populace alike becomes very clear. Prevention employing technology in our example could take the form of using a simple exercise machine to stay fit enough to keep walking along the familiar routes, to the library or club meeting, or to the store or the dance–thus the problem of mobility-related loneliness is prevented; it is never allowed to develop.

If, however, there were some reason that prevention of disability in walking didn't work, the person might want to try some form of compensation in the environment or the self, such as utilizing a cane. The person could also compensate for declining fitness by altering the transportation environment, maybe by obtaining a motor scooter or adopting some specialized aid for walking such as high tech shoes.

Even when we can't prevent the occurrence of a problem, can't compensate in order to eliminate it, then we can still help the providers of care. In gerontechnology we tend to view care as being assistance involving people. For instance, we might supply a medical technician to install special equipment and establish procedures for monitoring, or we might develop an informal network such as a telephone circle where a group of people would telephone each other cyclically everyday in some fixed order. In gerontechnology we concern ourselves less with the care itself and focus on providing technology to help the people who administer the care, including self care.

The last of the five aspects is research. It underlies each of the others. In the case of loneliness we might instigate psycho-pharmaceutical research into a mood elevator that is more suitable for the aging metabolism, one that doesn't have age related side effects, doesn't harm the person's liver or interact with other medicines that older people tend to use, and doesn't lead to dependence. Research is a broader concept that is used here as shorthand for the triad: research, development, and design, abbreviated as RD&D.

We simply employ the scientific method as we collect data and continue developing models and theories. Thus we can improve our conceptualizations both of the technologies that become available and of older people and sharpen our insights about how the two actually fit together.

On the high-tech side: Mathematical modeling and simulation

Older people's various situations can be overwhelming to human intuition depending on where along the continuum of complexity a situation falls. While it may be immediately obvious, from simply looking, that some person doesn't need a cane for walking, it isn't obvious precisely how much insulin to administer after a person of 80 kg and a height of 1.80 m has walked six kilometers at eight kilometers per hour on a hot day, consumed three grams of sugar one hour ago and been subjected to a host of other factors that make the glucose level go up and down. Similarly, it isn't obvious how much money will be saved in the long run by spending a specific amount of money on gerontechnological research in some future year, nor is it clear what effect the violet mercury vapor street lights have on a person's vision and ability to detect yellow curb markings or trip hazards, as a function of age.

Problems of this sort have been dealt with in many other fields by capitalizing on the fact that sets of mathematical equations can be developed that behave like specific physical systems, that behave like the body's hormonal systems do, behave like the results of expenditures on health care, like people walking. These can be used to model (act like) the systems of interest. They can be computerized and equipped with affable interfaces so that investigators can observe the simulated systems in action using the methods of scientific visualization. They can learn new things about the real system by performing "what if" tests on the model, can employ destructive testing without damage to anything, can predict the behavior of the system, and can devise and test ways of stabilizing it when it becomes unstable from too much blood sugar or from tripping or from draught in the fields. Virtually any bodily function can be modeled in relation to most of the factors that might affect it, as can social functions, mood, walking, air quality, driving, and even aging itself.
Chapter Seven is devoted to this powerful set of methods.

Consider an example of a database of the sort that lends itself to data mining and modeling. The National Agency for Welfare and Health of Finland has developed a software package for planning welfare and health services for older people (Hämäläinen & Vaarama, 1992). Workshops, interviews with experts, and brainstorming sessions led to a software-planning package consisting of a database of services for older people and four "planning models." The software allows the user to simulate alternative, functional future policies in the care of older people. The program can describe and analyze the current situation. It can function in short-term, medium-term, and long-term planning. It allows for systematic experiments with various models of the service system. It can accommodate the planning of various mixes of public and private sector involvement in service production.

Here, technology for computerization and mathematical modeling technology have been used to extend human capacities for assimilation of data and prediction of consequences for older people beyond normal human limits. For example, the database keeps track of some 200 variables related to welfare and health services. It includes 460 municipalities, 12 provinces, and the entire country. It has population projections up to the year 2030 from the Central Statistical Office.

As an added benefit, mathematical modeling of older people and their circumstances can lead directly to the invention and design of new technical aids, for instance personal instruments. "Sentient shoes" could anticipate and prevent many slips, trips, and falls. Canes, hats, athletic helmets, clothing, and portable devices with refined sensibilities, with awareness of global and local position, with links to knowledge bases and communications networks, with mnemonic and cognitive prostheses, offer older people many exciting possibilities through mathematical formulation and analysis.

Box 1.5 Misinterpretation of experimental results

Often it may seem necessary to compare older people with younger people along some dimension. For instance, it may be found that more automobile accidents of a certain type involve older people. Then it may be useful to determine whether some factor that is related to that specific type of accident is a factor that older people have trouble with. Reaction time, peripheral vision, or the digits or words that a person can remember from highway signs are a few of the factors that might be involved.

If experimentation determines that in fact there are more slow, or partially blind, or absent minded people among older people, the tendency is strong to "design for older people," redesign the highway, the car, or the task, or perhaps restrict the driving of older people. This is often a mistake. To illustrate, if all of the older people were taken off the road, for example, the dangerous younger people remaining in these categories of debilitation would still be driving. The accidents would continue, and the majority of the older people who are normal would be punished unnecessarily. Instead, we should focus our redesigning on the slow, the partially blind, and the absent minded (which each and every one of us in fact is at least part of the time) and leave the older people out of it. It stigmatizes them unfairly and leads to misconceptions of the actual issues in safety.

To illustrate with actual data, consider the two graphs.

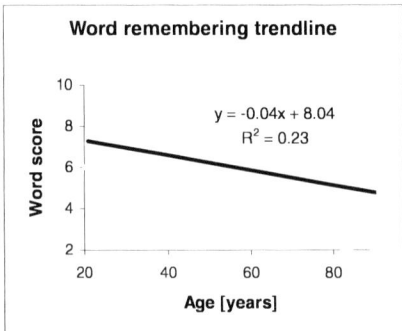 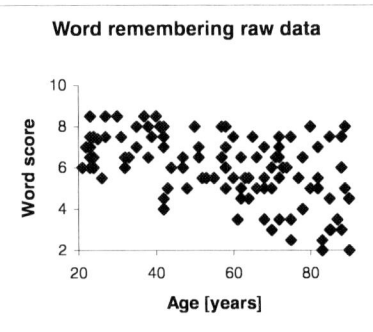

Figure 1 Data of an unpublished experiment on word remembering as a function of age; final result left graph, raw data right graph.

This is primarily based on data from an unpublished experiment–valuable information, but be very careful. Clearly there is a strong relation between age and the ability to remember words–or is there? What does such a relationship really mean? Where did it come from? Does your ability to remember words, or to react or to make decisions or figure things out or perform other tasks really decline with age so that we should simplify such tasks for older people?

Or is it simply that a few older people have developed problems and they pull the average down for older people in general? Part of the answer is evident from the second inset, which shows performance on this task as a function of age–this is the "raw" swarm-of-bees data underlying the straight-line relationship shown in the first inset.

"And now you know the rest of the story." Some in the group of older people were worse, which is what we would expect from small strokes, incipient Alzheimer's, and so forth. But, most individual data points from the older people can't be distinguished reliably from the twenty-year olds. Which all suggests that there may be no useable statement about the performance of individual older people in this data, none, just a statement about disease which may be a totally separate issue. Should we often simply be characterizing and designing for the lame, the specifically impaired, instead of for older people?

Let's take the issue of misinterpreting data on older people a bit further. Students in technical areas are accustomed to well-behaved data, to systems that actually behave like the straight-line summary of the data in the first inset. In cases where living matter is involved however, extreme variability in the data is common. Students in psychology and physiology are taught statistical methods for reformulating these clouds of bees.

The statistically unschooled reader would possibly see the correlation, represented by the line in the inset as implying a strong effect, assuming that the very strongest effect would only be –1.00. A more statistically sophisticated experimentalist would realize that only some 23% of the variance was related to age.

Two things combine in the data of the inset to give the appearance of strong correlation. First, there is a ceiling effect that skews the variability–people can easily get worse from trivial factors such as drowsiness whereas it is more difficult to become better. Second, the variability of the data increases with age for whatever reason, a common finding when age is involved. This makes any line fitted to the data to appear sloped, not because the older people are performing badly, but because a few of them are.

Most important in some ways, there are older people who are statistically indistinguishable from the very best of the young subjects, and there are young people who are worse than most of the older ones–one young person is below the median for those in their 90's. In the literature this situation is found often, together with the misinterpretation "People get worse when they get older." Often no raw data is presented, usually there is no standard error presented. There is sometimes a tendency to see the older people who are performing well as exceptions to the rule. Data, more carefully scrutinized, often shows the opposite–those older people who decline are exceptions, and rare ones at that. Beware!

Beware also of the effects of averaging the data points. The average obscures the extremes, the slowest, the dimmest, the people with the least acuity; yet these are the people, whether they be young or old, who are most likely to have the accidents, and for whom we should be designing.

Bailer, J.C. & Mosteller, F. (Eds.). (1986). Medical Uses of Statistics.
New England Journal of Medicine Books, Waltham, MA. ISBN 0-910133-16-6.

Low-tech: An example of an inventive technical solution

A good solution doesn't have to be mathematically derived, nor very highly technical, it just has to work well under the specific conditions without causing additional trouble. Having something to hold on to, or even just to touch as a perceptual reference, can allow a person to compensate for disorientation and perhaps prevent a fall, or can allow a person to rise from a sitting or lying position when they might not have been able to otherwise. However, it is nearly impossible to install rails or grab bars everywhere that they might be needed using standard methods. Fernie (1992) reports on a device, SturdyGrip™ that operates on the principle of a pole lamp. It is a vertical pole that can be placed anywhere in a room. It is held in place between the floor and the ceiling by compressive force. It can be positioned by the bed, in the bathroom, or beside a stairway to provide a reliable support to grasp for physical stability or perceptual reference. The poles can be used in combination with horizontal bars attached to them to act as guides, grab bars, or handrails. This is an innovation that is simple, low cost, effective, reversible, and modifiable. Yet, even this excellent device may need to be technically fortified for some applications because it requires a sturdy ceiling. The ever-dangerous bear's favor looms up once again because relying on any technology that fails can be worse than not having the technology at all.

Gerontechnology and the dimensions of aging

In theory at least, there is a vein of technology, known or unknown, which runs parallel to each of the veins of gerontology. To illustrate the distinction between the two fields, loss of hearing is gerontological, hearing aids are gerontechnological: diminished vision from glare due to aging lenses in the eye is in the province of gerontology, glasses matched with appropriately designed characteristics of optical transmission are gerontechnological. In general, for each decline along some dimension of aging, there is some technology that can be harnessed. Consider some of this parallel territory in relation to sensing, thinking and performing.

It is a fact of gerontology that sensory modalities may drift in specific ways with age. A modality is a subsystem of a "sense" as with the dimension or modality of pitch, high to low, in the sense of hearing. Other modalities are pain, hue, brightness, and pressure. Any modality can change with age, and most do, at least for some people. Any of the changes can cause undesirable effects, and if such effects affect aspects of daily living they are targets of gerontechnology. Then the modalities are enhanced, or alternate modalities are used to perform the affected tasks.

Hearing sensitivity

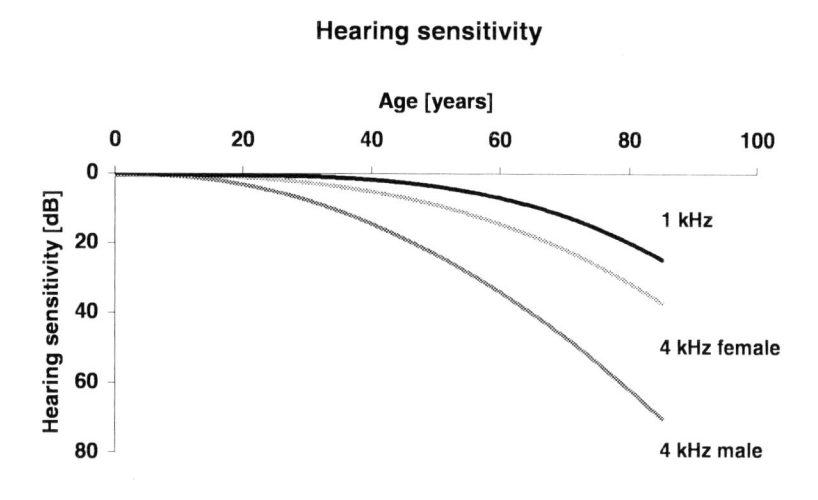

Figure 1.2 Thresholds for hearing as a function of age. Data from Scharf & Buus (1986).

An example of psychophysical characterizations of aging sensibilities is shown in Figure 1.2. Hearing thresholds as shown in the graph, averaged over the experimental population, fall off by on the order of 20 dB over the course of 80 years for 1 kHz tones. Sensitivity to 4 kHz tones, shown in the lower two curves for men and for women, is affected much more by age. For a 90-year-old male the extrapolated threshold dictates that for a 4 kHz sound to be heard it would need to be presented at the level of a jet aircraft. Elsewhere we note that modern electronic beepers deliver their peak energy at about this frequency and fall off rapidly as frequency decreases. They quite possibly won't be heard at all by older people with a hearing deficit.

Vibration threshold on the skin shows a similar falloff that is dependent on frequency, with the higher frequencies again being more affected.

The falloff in visual acuity, averaged over the experimental population, decreases progressively from about ten years of age to on the order of half of its original by age 90.

Often the problem in any of these cases is one of sharpening up the signal, providing a better signal to noise ratio, as opposed to simply increasing the intensity, which in extremes can even damage the sensory organ of older people. In vision higher contrast is sometimes more effective than higher luminance, which can also result in additional negative effects such as glare. Extensive work in psychophysics has been done to characterize these changes. But much more effort in gerontechnology needs to be made to relate the specifics of sensory change to the situations and tasks where they might cause problems.

Cognitive dimensions also are important. Clarity and quickness of thought, the ability to achieve realistic solutions, dimensions of awareness can all change with age, not necessarily for the worse. They have to be characterized experimentally, modeled and understood in relation to performance under specific circumstances of walking, driving, and performing other tasks.

The performance may drift along assorted dimensions too. Factors such as reaction time, allocation of attention, the informational processing times, time to complete a task, accuracy, endurance, and a hundred others enter into the safe timely functioning at home, on the highways, or at work. These may change with age, again perhaps for the better, perhaps not. Gerontechnology looks for ways to assess and maintain the levels of performance that are necessary to keep people who are becoming older, competitive and safe.

Accidents, technology, and safety

Older people are of course subjected to most of the same factors that cause accidents among the young so they experience the same slips, trips, falls, wrecks, injuries from sports and other damaging experiences. In general, older people function very well in the world in circumstances that are dangerous to everyone, as pedestrians, drivers, skiers, joggers, and swimmers. But there are some problems that require our attention.

First their vulnerabilities are somewhat different. They may withstand a specific accident well, or not, both as a function of age and in terms of their individual characteristics. Many older people are more frangible; they break easily. Some are so fragile that in a fall their bones break from sheer muscle tension before they hit the ground, some retinas may detach more easily, and so on. The annual litigation costs in the U.S.A. for hip fractures are on the order of a billion (1,000,000,000) dollars. Try to estimate roughly how much of this money one of your hypothetical solutions, such as a miniature airbag, could save.

Second, designers who are concerned about safety in public places don't ordinarily design specifically for old age. They are concerned with the entire panorama of human disabilities. So they simply must design for the worst possible cases, for the people who may have problems with vision, ambulation, and so on. This has the effect of automatically including older people who do have these same problems. Nevertheless, gerontechnology needs to monitor the standards that are set to be sure that the older people are included properly, and aren't harmed by safety standards developed for the younger people or the handicapped. For example, in lighting the young may require a certain level of lighting for reading warnings or for walking along a pathway at night. Older people might require additional light too. But if the light were not positioned well away from the axis of sight, if it were "shining in the eyes," the older people with their elevated vulnerabilities to glare could be blinded by it.

Third, the hypothetical worst-case older victim faces a formidable array of situations that the young don't usually have to deal with. The lessened sensory acuities, diminished coordination, balance, and modes of recovery put them in danger in ordinary situations where normal people, young or old, may be fairly safe. These include a host of otherwise non-threatening hazards such as walking through leaves, turning around in the shower and walking or standing in accelerating buses.

Fourth, some older people find themselves in new potentially hazardous situations that the young usually aren't subjected to, such as having to change modes of locomotion altogether. For instance, for a few, this may involve the dangerous feat of getting into and out of a wheel chair, or walking on crutches or with a cane or walker, each with its own sets of challenges. Similarly, bifocals cause deceptive impressions of distances.

Each bit of assistive technology designed to help may bring with it its own sets of dangers. Ironically, much of the common equipment recommended at a typical hospital for hip fracture patients when they are discharged carries the danger of getting in the way of normal functioning and precipitating an accident. These implements include walkers, long-handled sponges, new tub equipment (e.g. a stool, which may then be tripped over), rolling carts, canes or quad canes that are in themselves tripping hazards.

Sometimes certain types of fluorescent lighting may be unpleasant for older people. As often happens, in lighting the highway we have two separate factors that can converge for older people. On the one hand, visual sensitivity declines so that it may be more difficult to see an appropriate distance ahead of the car at night. Second, reaction to road hazards may be slowed with age. Thus older people may see problems arising more unexpectedly than when they were young, and aggravating the situation they may respond to the problems later. This in turn means that they may have to slam on the brakes at the last minute, creating a dangerous situation for the driver behind. With lighting designed for older eyes the problem would be minimal, without specialized lighting it is severe.

Because of literally hundreds of factors such as these, throughout this book we will continually be returning to the issue of safety in an assortment of contexts, in housing, with respect to mathematical modeling and prediction of danger, in traffic, with respect to ambulation, in simulation of debilitating conditions, and with respect to personal instruments that can be used to lessen the chances of accidents.

A historical note

Of course, throughout history, many technical groups have applied their technology to specific problems of older people. But this activity usually has been performed in a crisis-driven mode dealing mainly with serious and imminent problems related to the care of the sickly aged. The solutions often came from medical or assistive technologies. As we have noted, gerontechnology is unique by virtue of its deliberate comprehensiveness. The actual term, gerontechnology, was coined at the Eindhoven University of Technology (Graafmans & Brouwers, 1989). This name supplemented an existing term, "Technology and Aging," which is still used and for our purposes here was roughly parallel. Bouma (1992), in an article in the first book devoted to the new field, per se, at the time provided the first publicized definition of gerontechnology as being, "the study of technology and aging for the improvement of the daily functioning of the elderly." He pointed out that the terms Technology, and Aging, in the context of ergonomics, then and still now, are intended as very encompassing designations including research, design, and development, manufacture and marketing.

Now a number of formal groups at universities, especially throughout Europe, North America, and in Japan, have formed under the rubric of gerontechnology. There are international conferences and governmental funding has been developed in a number of countries. For example, COST A5, a Europe-wide network for planning and investigating issues related to older people was established by the governments of European countries. The findings of this group indicated that specific training and education were needed to produce researchers dedicated to this new field. The objective of this training will be to make them aware of the age-related changes in human functioning and to train them in translating knowledge about the aging process and about the aspirations and desires of older people into appropriate products, technologies, and systems.

This type of activity defines the major goals for education in gerontechnology: first, creation of a knowledge base of principles, methods and facts about aging and technology, and second, creation of an "attitude base" bearing on the convictions, beliefs, and goals of society.
This book was written to support these needs.
In the next chapters, we will concentrate on vital aspects of older people's life: health (Chapter 2), housing (Chapter 3), working (Chapter 4), mobility (Chapter 5), and communication (Chapter 6). Chapter 7 deals with the methodology of mathematical modeling as a research tool. Chapter 8 is a concluding chapter that also is intended as an outlook toward the near future.

Suggested readings

Birren, J.E. & Schaie, K.W. (Eds.). (1995). Handbook of the psychology of aging. 4th Edition. Academic Press, San Diego. ISBN 0-122-101261-1.

Bouma, H. (1992). Gerontechnology: Making technology relevant for the elderly. In: H. Bouma & J.A.M. Graafmans. (Eds.). Gerontechnology. Proceedings of the first International Conference on Gerontechnology, Eindhoven, August 1991. (pp. 1-5). IOS Press, Amsterdam. ISBN 90-5199-072-3.

Fisk, A.D. & Rogers, W.A. (Eds.). (1996). Handbook of human factors and the older adult. Academic Press, San Diego. ISBN 0-12-257680-2.

Graafmans, J., Taipale, V. & Charness, N. (Eds.). (1998). Gerontechnology: A sustainable investment in the future. Proceedings of the second International Conference on Gerontechnology, Helsinki, October 1996. IOS Press, Amsterdam. ISBN 90-5199-367-6.

Spirduso, W.W. (1995). Physical dimensions of aging. Human Kinetics, Champaign, IL, USA. ISBN 0-87322-323-3.

Suggested websites

http://statline.cbs.nl/statweb/index.stm
The statistical database on the Netherlands. [in Dutch]

http://www.aarp.org
Website of the American Association of Retired Persons, a non-profit organization for older people.

http://www.eurolinkage.org
Website of Eurolink Age, a network of organizations and individuals that promotes good policy and practice on aging in the interests of the 121 million older people in the European Union.

http://www.gerontechnology.org
Website of the International Society for Gerontechnology.

http://www.nidi.nl
Website of the Netherlands Interdisciplinary Demographic Institute.

http://www.un.org/esa/socdev/ageing.htm
United Nation's Aging site.

CHAPTER TWO

Healthy Aging

Introduction

Maintaining the options of older people by preventing threats to health, and even by challenging the aging process itself, is a fundamental concern of gerontechnology. Doing this involves several arms of technology. Diagnostic technologies are needed to monitor physiological states and to screen for disorders of the body's systems and internal organs. Efforts in food technology provide roads to optimal nutrition that vary with age–for instance, the parameters of digestion change. More information about the effects of diet is needed that focuses on older people. The technology of sports and exercise provides information about the effects of activity on older people and dictates ways of stimulating and regulating physical effort and exercise. And the fruits of research in the basic sciences, especially biology and chemistry, often metamorphose into technologies that suit and serve the physiological well being of older people.

Why is there growing reason for concern?

There are several reasons that it is becoming more pressing to develop preventive measures and techniques of human replenishment. Pushing life expectancy upward as we presently are doing necessarily grants more time to the diseases of wear and tear for grinding away at each of us at our many points of bodily vulnerability. Also, there are more of us in the ranks of the worn and torn. According to the World Health Organization (1998), the average life expectancy at birth in 1955 was just 48 years. In 2025 it will reach 73 years. Many of the babies born this day will welcome the 22nd century. There were only 200 centenarians in France in 1950.
In the year 2050 the projection is for an increase of nearly 1,000 fold (actually 750) to 150,000.

Most of these figures are simple extrapolations of the numbers. It is impossible to predict breakthroughs of course, but if progress in medical technology is also extrapolated then the projections become far more extreme.

An additional reason for the increasing importance of technology to health as we age is that age per se makes us more easy to abrade by circulatory, respiratory, and cancer's families of diseases. Cancer and heart disease are most threatening to people in the 70 to 75 age group. This means, on the positive side, that when you become older than 75 these diseases won't be quite as menacing to you statistically. But you will be more prone to impairments of hearing, vision, mobility, and mental functioning after 75.

Relevant to this, the age group that has been growing faster in numbers than any of the others is that of people 85 and older, whose numbers have almost tripled to around 4 million in the U.S. since 1960. (Of course, the group is expanding upwards in age whereas the other groups can't by definition.) Still, the proportion of chronically disabled older Americans has fallen steadily in the past decade. People are in better shape and they feel good too apparently. Most people 50 and older say that they feel at least 15 years younger than their chronological age.

Governments are beginning to appreciate the need for special applications of technology. As a report by the European Commission in 1996 phrased it, "With increasing life expectancy of older people, disabilities and chronic disease ... need special attention. They include physical disabilities such as joint diseases, sensory disabilities, including poor hearing, and mental disabilities such as dementia."

In this chapter we will first examine the general layout of technology's foci in health as we consider the areas where the problems, from social to molecular, can be found. Then we will look at some of the technology in action, by way of example.

Overview of gerontechnology in the context of health and fitness

The regions where we presently need to work against the general deconditioning of people are depicted in Figure 2.1.

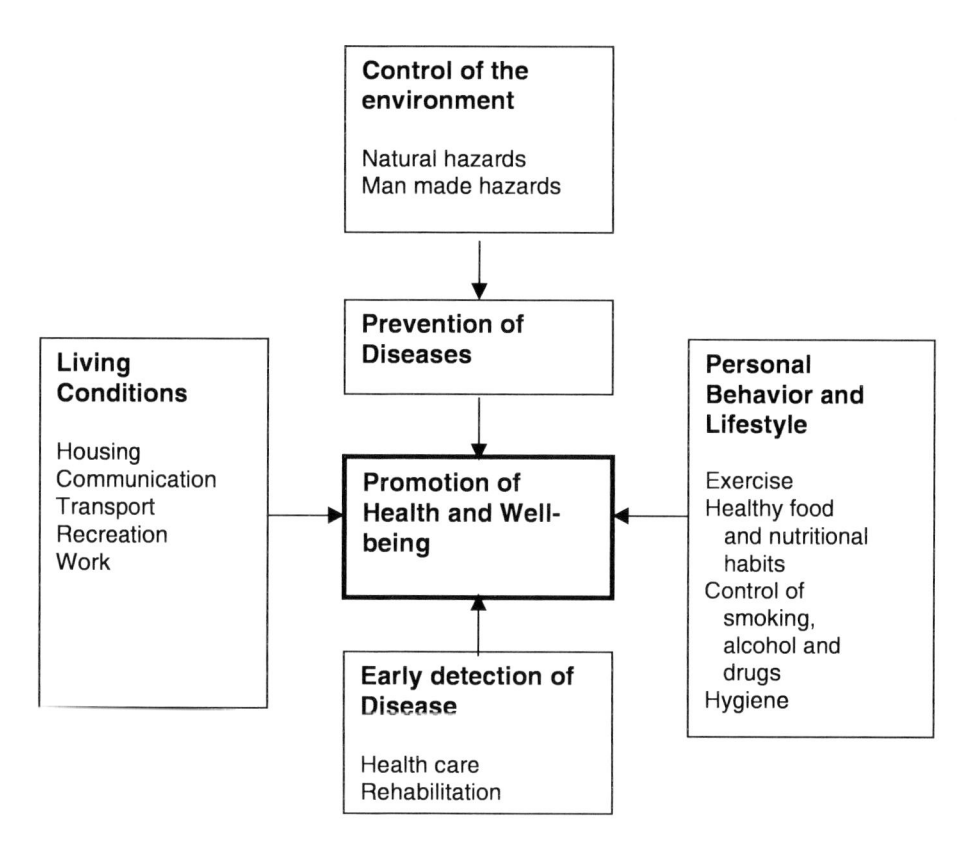

```
                    ┌─────────────────┐
                    │ Control of the  │
                    │ environment     │
                    │                 │
                    │ Natural hazards │
                    │ Man made hazards│
                    └────────┬────────┘
                             ↓
                    ┌─────────────────┐
┌──────────────┐    │ Prevention of   │    ┌──────────────┐
│ Living       │    │ Diseases        │    │ Personal     │
│ Conditions   │    └────────┬────────┘    │ Behavior and │
│              │             ↓             │ Lifestyle    │
│ Housing      │    ┌─────────────────┐    │              │
│ Communication│───▶│ Promotion of    │◀───│ Exercise     │
│ Transport    │    │ Health and Well-│    │ Healthy food │
│ Recreation   │    │ being           │    │   and nutritional│
│ Work         │    └────────▲────────┘    │   habits     │
│              │             │             │ Control of   │
│              │    ┌─────────────────┐    │   smoking,   │
│              │    │ Early detection │    │   alcohol and│
│              │    │ of Disease      │    │   drugs      │
│              │    │                 │    │ Hygiene      │
│              │    │ Health care     │    │              │
└──────────────┘    │ Rehabilitation  │    └──────────────┘
                    └─────────────────┘
```

Figure 2.1 Overview of regions for the promotion of health.

Referring to the top of Figure 2.1, first, by controlling and modifying the natural environment we can hope to banish certain specters of disease that typically hover over aging people. We can develop technology to eliminate contact with environmental contaminants, both natural and man-made. Natural hazards might include bacteria such as E-coli in the food and water supply, which we can eliminate by better filtering, sterilization and by monitoring parameters such as the coliform count. (The absence of coliform bacteria in drinking water is regarded as technology's certification of safety from any pathogenic bacteria in that sample of water.) Our own contributions can be controlled by avoiding the release of contaminant agents such as mercury of which 10,000 tons are produced and disappear annually into thermometers, instruments, chemicals, and the surroundings. The development of industrial standards appropriate to the very young and the very old are important here and they are possible. Dioxins, toxic to people, are released when chlorinated organic compounds such as some glues that go into materials for the construction of houses, particleboard, are burned. The present emission restrictions for dioxins in the emissions of new plants that turn household garbage into energy by burning it, in Sweden, is the approximate equivalent in terms of volume of putting half of the sugar you put into your morning coffee into Loch Ness Lake.

These environmental technologies join with medical technologies for the prevention of diseases such as diphtheria, exemplified by inoculation. Technology cleans up the environment, but the person is fortified too, just in case.

On the personal side, to the right in Figure 2.1, are things that technology can help older people themselves to do. It can help them maintain healthy lifestyles by assisting them with exercise and eating right and even, using artifacts such as "the patch," to avoid smoking and perhaps overindulgence in alcohol and harmful drugs.

The attendant factors to the left, factors of housing, communication, transportation, recreation, and work are aspects of the person's immediate environment. These moderate the rest of the scenario, variously helping the persons, or hindering them.

Technology has armaments to deal with the diseases and other problems that do get past the preventive measures of environmental control, inoculation and personal style. If diseases do get a foothold they can be vanquished more quickly if they are detected immediately. If this fails then we still have the technology of health care, including rehabilitation.

Box 2.1 Public Health Engineering

Public health engineering, originating as early as the 1880's, was originally intended as a line of defense against infectious diseases that were virtually decimating entire populations. Now our agencies of public health dwell on a broader spectrum of problems touching on issues ranging from social welfare to the spread of the common cold.

The current upheaval of technology will continue to increase both the power and the flexibility of public health. New devices and principles, miniaturization, and advances in computerization and mathematical modeling will be changing the technological picture dramatically.

Gerontechnology lives at the crossroads of advancing technology and advancing age. Accordingly, the task will be to provide a cadre of specialists who are educationally prepared to match the technology to the dimensions and nuances of the aging population. At this point we can realistically envision a field that could be entitled "Gerontechnology in Public Health Engineering."

Possibilities for careers for this new brand of engineer/scientist would include the following.

1. Scientific research in the interdisciplinary field of preventive technology and gerontechnology. For example, informatics, telematics, and domotics.
2. Participation in construction, design, and evaluation of products, processes, services, taking the issues of interfacing into consideration, hands on or through advisory groups.
3. Design and evaluation of environments for working with respect to prevention of problems.
4. Developing systems for physical, physiological, and behavioral monitoring and integrating them into the life fabric of people who may be at risk.
5. Supplying advice to public health and home care specialists.
6. Combining the economic aspects with issues of health, technology, and the environment.

http://www.gerontechnology.nl/phee.htm

The panorama of technology

Technology has been brought to bear on issues of protection for years, and we have relatively low-tech shields against unwanted energies everywhere. Throughout history we have devised technology for protecting ourselves against abrasion, particles, chemicals, light, contusions, and even the vacuum of outer space and the pressures of the deep with devices ranging from loin cloths and moccasins to space suits. What is being done to deal with problems of aging? Presently there is a search going on for technology to protect us at the molecular levels, for instance against free radicals. Hormones such as insulin become less effective with age and too much sugar in the blood can ravage us. Other molecules can too.

Molecules of aging, a chemical hypothesis

Oxidative stress simply means that structures within the body are subject to oxidation. Oxidation may be caused by oxygen, per se, (for instance, the oxygen molecules in the air challenge us "oxidatively" beginning with our first breaths) or oxidation may be caused by molecules that act chemically in the same way that oxygen does–they grab electrons from molecules. For historical reasons, electron borrowing is called oxidation even though no oxygen is involved.

To elaborate slightly, the atoms and molecules that we are made from are most stable when they possess their preferred numbers of electrons, in pairs. When an atom or molecule has an unpaired electron exposed to the world it is a "free radical." Free radicals are strongly predisposed to borrowing or sharing electrons with some other atom or molecule to reach their preferred quotas. Because of this over-eagerness, chemical reactions may take place that weren't supposed to according to the normal scheme, destroying the biochemical order and sometimes destroying molecules of body tissue and thus the cells.

To gain some appreciation for the seriousness of this, consider the types of cell and the cellular functions that are susceptible to damage and interference. They include DNA replication, which means that cells can't reproduce themselves correctly. Free radicals can be soluble in lipids so that they enter membranes and other parts of cells, nerves, muscles and organs and damage them. They can alter the genes that are blueprints for the manufacture of enzymes, which in turn manufacture the proteins that make up our tissues and perform other essential functions. Then the proteins may not work as well, or at all. Free radicals can initiate damaging chain reactions, grabbing electrons from one molecule, which in turn must snatch new electrons from somewhere else, creating cascades of imbalance and discord. Why don't these chemical processes immediately turn us into formless pools of oxidized protoplasm because of all of this potential destruction? Why don't we age instantly, lose our structures, wrinkle, falter, and wilt?

We have protective systems to stop aging–but they age

According to the theory, fortunately there are protective enzymes that are pulled into reactions and are themselves oxidized saving other vulnerable molecules from it. In addition, when there is damage and a strand of DNA or some other important entity is altered, there are repair molecules that can fix things back up the way they were.
Unfortunately the reserves of retaliation and repair become thinner with time. Our protective enzymes that soak up free radicals aren't as plentiful as they once were, our repair mechanisms aren't either, and both may be damaged. One damaged gene means one damaged enzyme that begins making its protein wrong, or not at all, or otherwise failing.

The fact that the very entities, which protect us from aging, age themselves is ironic and unsettling. However, there are indications that our front lines of defense can be rejuvenated. If this is true, then it is an issue for younger people. These effects can be cumulative–they may accumulate every second all throughout life, homing in on us more and more as our vulnerability rises simply because of the mounting damage.
Research into the contribution of free radicals to aging has very promising horizons. For example, presently some endogenous markers are known; one is antipyrine that allows us to assess how much oxidative stress is taking place in a person. This allows experimentation into ways of monitoring and controlling oxidative stress.

Hostile oxidative molecules have been subdued in similar areas in the past. Consider the classical case of blood glucose.

Box 2.2 Management of diabetes

As an illustration of the challenge to technology that corrections to the human mechanisms pose, consider some of the individual problems that must be overcome in the development of an insulin pump.

- The moment-to-moment need for insulin must be measured continuously, day and night. Presently, on the order of three billion dollars per year is spent on glucose monitoring strips, but these don't provide continuous monitoring. But, devices that can monitor continuously are presently being developed and approved for use and pumps will soon incorporate them. The technology of monitoring is proceeding in three directions. Non-invasive devices that don't require breaking the skin are under development. Probes can be placed under the skin now, but presently they require replacement in a matter of days. Devices that are available now can be surgically implanted that transmit glucose levels to external devices. These can last for several years.
- The ideal pump probably is one that can be implanted within the body. Presently this technology is being tested. It will be autonomous so that the user is free to sleep late on weekends, eat normally, and forget the device entirely.
- External pumps have reservoirs that must be filled with insulin from time to time. Filling the reservoirs of internal pumps requires that the skin be pierced.
- Reliability is a major issue. Severe damage can be done to the user within a few hours if the systems fail. Dual computers, sensory feedback, alarms, self-testing by the pump along most of its dimensions of operation are important. However, high voltage changes such as lightning nearby, van der Graaff generators and Tesla coils still could disable many of the safety measures.
- In addition to the "basal" flow of insulin, the pump or the user must monitor activities such as exercise and eating and inject "boluses" of insulin to offset these activities. Presently the user must plan and supervise this regime.

- Where should the insulin be applied? Injecting under the skin means that the insulin must travel through the blood stream to reach its site of action. Then it goes to organs that may suffer from it. Infusing into the interperitoneal cavity avoids this to some extent because more insulin goes to the liver. Other possible sites of application, each offering advantages and disadvantages are oral and nasal.
- Certain kinds of insulin won't work with some pumps. For example, insulin may not be compatible with the material in the tubing.
- Ideally, insulin with different rates of action is needed for different types of correction of blood sugar. Slow action stabilizes the system and removes dangerous peaks, but faster action is needed to correct quickly for factors such as exercise and then quickly disappear from the system so that the basal levels won't be affected.
- Pumps clog up. If a pump clogs, blood sugar can rise abruptly in only three or four hours leading quickly to the damaging state of ketoacidosis because, unlike with an injection, there is no pool of slower acting insulin under the skin.
- Pumps can leak, which is difficult for them to automatically detect.
- For diabetes that is caused by failed cells in the pancreas; perhaps it would be easier to solve the problem of pumping by using natural "pumps." Even now we can simply replace the cells that make insulin in the pancreas–put in new ones. However, beta cell replacement itself has some major problems. For example, these cells are very delicate and it is difficult to remove them from the donor pancreas without damaging them. It is necessary to find material to surround the cells with so that the recipient's immune system won't destroy them, and beta cells don't replace themselves so cells must be repeatedly transplanted.

An ominous molecule–sugar

Similar to the predatory activity of oxygen free radicals just discussed, glucose in the blood can randomly attach itself to sites on proteins and nucleic acid such as DNA in detrimental ways that are progressively harmful as we age. This is a major reason why diabetes is so damaging when it isn't checked. In the words of Spirduso (1995), "…the random attachment of proteins and the development of large tangles of malfunctioning molecules lead to many of the problems and systems that are associated with aging: stiffening of tissue, rigidity of blood vessels, tight ligaments and muscle tendons, cataracts, atherosclerosis and many more." In previous years there was scant hope for any victim of adult onset diabetes, which attacks a very large percentage of older people, sometimes causing blindness and a number of other afflictions. Now there is hope.

The hormone insulin modulates glucose levels. Hormones are chemical molecules that are secreted inside the body and carried about widely to affect distant organs. Of course, insulin now can be injected or otherwise administered to cause the removal of glucose, so dangerous to tissue cells, from the blood stream.

Pause for a moment to appreciate the array of side-technologies that had to be developed, evaluated, and delivered to the market in order to allow a diabetic in these modern times to self-test blood sugar and administer corrective insulin.

A good example of the application of technology to diabetes is WellMate. This system for the telematic management of diabetes was unveiled at the 16th International Diabetes Federation Congress in Helsinki in 1997. The concept aims at providing a flexible and easy-to-use system for daily monitoring of information related to an individual's diabetic state. It also allows low cost communication between the persons and the physician. This is the first-ever wireless tool for health care for diabetics. The measurement and control system enabled by WellMate is based on a digital cellular phone, which is used to collect and transmit the blood glucose value and other data related to the diabetic's state to a database on a daily basis. The data is automatically analyzed and formatted so that authorized physicians and the patient can have access to the results, either over the digital cell phone or over the Internet!

Because it has recently been discovered that maintaining more rigid control over glucose levels can slow down or even prevent the development of the standard problems, one goal of this system is to allow the individual to be able to learn to apply tighter control.

Challenges to technology in the physical administering of insulin.

Each day some 1700 new cases of diabetes are diagnosed in the U.S.A. Of Americans, around forty percent of those with diabetes are using insulin. As people age, their tendencies to become diabetic increase so the delivery of insulin is a major issue among older people.

Now that the metabolic relationships between insulin and glucose are known, countering the problem would seem to be a simple technological problem: monitor blood sugar and infuse insulin accordingly into the blood stream. However, it seems that when human physiology is involved that application of technology is never simple even though the actual problem itself may seem to be. Early artificial hearts "bruised" the blood, broke the platelets and made it clot. Gentle peristaltic pumps can be used in the operating room, but are at the moment too large and power hungry to be implanted permanently. New joints can be implanted but some of the materials can be foci of microorganisms.

One wonders, with such technology and the control that it offers, is all of this molecular devastation we have discussed thus far avoidable, or is that just a dream? Is disaster built inextricably into our cells and their environments? Even if it is, perhaps it is avoidable. Sperm cells replicate endlessly without mistakes and red blood cells and some cells in the gut seem to be less susceptible. True, our chromosomes are different, but since the human system works at all it may, possibly with a bit of help from the right technology, be able to work flawlessly.

Box 2.3 Telomeres: The fuses of aging?

Theories of aging seem inexhaustible. They focus on molecular ravaging of various kinds, on chemical destruction, immune deficiencies, all varieties of stress, cross-linked collagen costing us our elasticity, diet, and spontaneous mutations in the genetic mechanisms of the cells. Now new evidence on genetic involvement in aging is indicating that there are specific structures called telomeres on both ends of the chromosomes that erode a little with each reproduction just like small fuses on fire crackers burning down. Eventually there is no more telomere material left and the erosion begins to operate on the genetic material itself. It has been found when replicating human cells that it can only be done a certain number of generations, called the Hayflick number. Perhaps there is a relationship. The chromosome duplication of cell reproduction may stop when the telomere is gone, or be carried out incorrectly, or the raw endings of chromosomes may connect to each other. It is suggestive that an enzyme, telomerase, is able to rebuild the telomeres. Even more suggestive, our immortal cells: germ cells (which give rise to eggs and sperm) and cancer cells seem to be able to produce telomerase. If this enzyme were made available to all of our cells, would we still age? (There has been some thought about making cancer cells age more rapidly by depriving them of telomerase, but preliminary experimentation with mice indicates that the mechanisms of cancer may not necessarily depend critically on telomerase.) Unfortunately, at this point even after all of this research we don't know why we age. Are we perhaps simply trying to track down an enemy, Age, that doesn't really exist as a single creature?

Medina, J.J. (1996). The clock of ages: why we age, how we age, winding back the clock. Cambridge University Press, Cambridge. ISBN 0-521-46244-4.

Orchestrating a healthy lifestyle

There are some very simple things that older people and we, who are presently auditioning to join older people, can be educated to do. For instance, the ability to defend against free radicals is thought to be related to lifestyle. For example, smoking has been implicated. Hormones such as insulin, and our enzymes that manufacture us and then protect us are involved, and the hormone adrenaline, which pervades our lives and feelings when we are stressed, can create surpluses of oxygen and glucose.

Diet

It may seem counterintuitive in a sense that diet could be very critically important. Our systems have such vast reserves. It is hard to imagine that a carrot or cabbage or a small capsule of gooey liquid with a few molecules in it would be more than a drop in the ocean of a human with trillions of free radical reactions taking place constantly, reactions that are being effectively dealt with. In fact, such very small amounts of chemicals are effective because many similar molecules are already in place doing their jobs. When a molecule of antioxidant floats past a membrane that already has plenty of similar protective molecules and there are no workplaces open, nothing happens and it floats on by. But when it floats into a region with a deficit, for some reason not enough protectors showed up for work, it is pulled into service. The molecules in the capsule or the carrot aren't going to be the main contingent, they are the reserves.

Helpful diets and supplements can affect older people more than the young partly because their assorted reserves may become less vast. So can destructive commodities such as alcohol, nicotine, and other drugs affect them more? For one thing, these are thought to increase the numbers of free radicals. The adage is, "One cigarette requires 25 milligrams of vitamin C." An orange on the tree has around 50 milligrams, and after it sits around for a few days its content is down around 25.
Extrapolating our exemplar hypothesis of free radicals into the arena of diet, uric acid, glutathionine, ascorbic acid, vitamin E, beta-carotene and a number of other chemicals are "antioxidants." Since these molecules can deal with free radicals and can go where the action is and police it, according to theory they may thus help keep us young.
But, a healthy lifestyle is a multidimensional tightrope.

If you lean too far to the right, you fall; too much to the left and you fall too, and the balance point changes with age. As an example, vitamin A may be able to protect us, but it is also poisonous in large amounts because our systems can't dissolve it with water and flush it out–we can't eat livers from polar bear. In contrast, vitamin C is water-soluble, so it can perform inside the cells and fluid bodies, and our systems can flush it out with water if there is too much.

A word of caution is possibly appropriate. The free radical hypothesis, appealing though it may be for simple dietary guidance–don't eat too many things that are oxidized, eat plenty of antioxidants–is only under test. Presently, though we have accumulated a great deal of knowledge about the relation of anti-oxidants and free radicals in our systems, more field studies are needed and from our point of view in gerontechnology, much additional testing will have to focus the results that are forthcoming onto the metabolism of older people. The search for other things that age us is continuing along many avenues. Consider the case of our bones.

Another side of nutrition

In some extreme cases, long term biochemical cause and effect have been worked out because they are striking and obvious. We know about many of the major poisons because they have quick and dramatic effects. We have learned not to eat the leaf blades in rhubarb with their ethanedioic acid and we don't eat hemlock. We know what to eat to prevent scurvy because the symptoms are so severe. We even know a little about subtle effects of cholesterol. But the more subtle diseases, the slower ones, those that age us insidiously over many years, and the poisons that are slow and cumulative have probably for the most part evaded us.

One triumph in preventive technology is related to the discovery of osteoporosis advancing on the bones of older people slowly and quietly, undetected–until a bone breaks. Now we have arrived at some tentative facts about replenishing bone density with calcium to save our aging hips– and we realized that vitamin D is necessary to assure that the calcium pills we take in fact end up on our bones. Estrogen replacement therapy and the newer medications that increase bone density are perhaps even more significant. Technology hopefully will be able to decrease the costs of production and promote wider distribution, administration, and testing.

Box 2.4 Gender differences in health

According to the World Health Organization's research report for 1998, women make up the majority of the older population in virtually all countries. Women have different circumstances, challenges, and health concerns than men as they age. The major issues of their health center around cardiovascular disease and stroke, cancers, musculoskeletal conditions such as arthritis and osteoporosis, neurological or mental disorders, degenerative disorders such as losses in vision and hearing, and chronic obstructive pulmonary disease. A paramount health challenge is to postpone or treat these conditions.

In the United States, 55% of women over 75 with coronary heart disease are disabled by their illness. Breast cancer costs women 10 years of life expectancy whereas cancer of the prostate reduces the average life expectancy of men by only one year. Lung cancer has overtaken breast cancer in women of the United States, in conjunction with their rise in smoking, and the pattern is spreading to women elsewhere, although quitting smoking is one of the most easily accessible preventive measures.

Musculoskeletal conditions can be offset in many cases by exercise. Yet few older women exercise on a regular basis in developed countries. Lack of exercise and inappropriate nutrition have led to an increase in the proportion of women who are overweight or obese. In contrast, in developing countries too much exercise in a sense is part of the problem. Dealing with heavy loads leads to damage of the joints. In developing countries, under-nutrition is a problem among the oldest of old women. Osteoporosis and the associated fractures cause huge medical expense, both monetary and physical. And it is estimated that the number of hip fractures could rise from 1.7 million in 1990 to around 6.3 million by 2050. Women represent 80% of those who have hip fractures. Women are more prone because their loss of bone accelerates after the menopause.

Prevention is possible with hormone therapy, but that may make them susceptible to other diseases such as breast cancer. Between 30 and 40 women out of every 100 will experience an osteoporotic fracture, compared to 13 men.

World Health Organization. (1998). The World Health Report. Life in the 21st century: a vision for all. World Health Organization, Geneva. ISBN 92-4-156189-0.

Physical exercise

Recent research indicates that the implications of moderate physical exercise go far beyond the hardening of muscles and the conditioning of the heart and lungs that we have come to associate it with. Exercise can be good or bad in very idiosyncratic ways. It appears that it is important to design exercise equipment with muscle-by-muscle envelopes of overexertion in mind.

On one hand, there is research that suggests some ominous effects of too much exercise of a muscle: during exercise oxygen free radicals are released because of oxidative phosphorylation in the mitochondria of muscle cells, their energy centers, and from inflammatory cells, which may enhance events that impinge on the antioxidant defenses. As age increases, the balance between the oxidizers and the protectors apparently becomes more sensitive to physical stress. So, one possible conclusion is that older people are more susceptible to oxidative muscle damage from physical activity (Meydani, 1992).

However, daily physical exercise is positive as a rule, including exercise of the muscles, and the heart and lungs. But the amount seems to need careful monitoring and apportioning, perhaps at the level of the individual muscle. The modern tools for toning are specialized machines, treadmills, grip strengtheners, rowing machines, which are specialized for individual muscle groups, but these are still fairly blunt instruments. We need machines that can provide more specific tailoring to the range of problems that develop over the age span.

The biochemical interactions are complex, but one tentative implication is this. In older people the balance between the production of free radicals caused by exercising, and the compensatory increases in ability to deal with free radicals that exercise provides, may be tilted in favor of the free radicals. Thus it may be that those older people who exercise should take antioxidants. Still, even if the theme of oxidation is totally true, and it may not be, an incredible amount of work still needs to be done to allow us to tell any specific older person, or even older people in general, whether and how to exercise with respect to only this one simple dimension of concern.

The role of gerontechnology and science

Just as the molecular processes in the body discover food, bring it into the body to nourish the cells, reshape it and catalyze its actions, we nourish the movement, gerontechnology, by foraging for and feeding it scientific discoveries and research old and new which we then bring together in the field and in laboratories and catalyze into actions that benefit older people.

But isn't the work that is being done now by scientists already optimally functional for older people, even if only because it is motivated by the scientist's awareness of his/her own aging? Isn't it automatically oriented at least to some extent toward problems of older people? Not necessarily. There may be plenty of special food for your geriatric hound on the shelves of your supermarket, but there is probably less for older people, even less for special categories of older people and for older women.
We have plenty of scientists. But in many cases they need to be made aware of the parameters of older people so that they can be included in the research.

The largest international chemical society alone has well over 150,000 members, many of whom understand and manipulate atoms on a daily basis, which are associated with problems and processes underlying aging, nutrition, and health. On the order of ten thousand new chemicals are reported every week or so. The doctors and medical students in the American Medical Association (AMA) number 300,000 and the largest American Dietetic Association (ADA) has 70,000 members spread over 28 subspecialties. Another 40,000 people belong to the Physical Society, and the American Mathematical Society alone has another 20,000 members.

Given the present explosion of science, given the number of scientists working on the problems, wouldn't you think that any and all new discoveries immediately would be passed on to older people?
Without meaning to overlook what science has accomplished for us already, we should note that the process of science proceeds slowly on its own driven more by considerations of funding than considerations of need. It requires foraging and catalysis and guidance if older people are to be served well. Consider an example.

Many studies have been conducted and many are in progress, for example, using animal models to determine the effects of a very wide range of dietary modifications on longevity (Ausman & Russell, 1990). However, do the regulatory agencies need to be made more sensitive to older people? For instance, should they at least be expected to specify the ages of test animals if not include age as a variable? Shouldn't gender, which becomes more important with age along some dimensions, also be reported?

Box 2.5 Research misses the aging

Pigs are commonly used as biomedical research models in many problems that are close to the concerns of the older people. For example, these include cardiovascular research, atherosclerosis, obesity, and susceptibility to stressing agents and gastrointestinal diseases. Pigs are models for diabetes, alcoholism, and ulcers. They have been used to study melanomas and reactivity of the skin to actinic rays. They are used to test for toxic effects of chemicals and in questions of nutrition. The difficulty of generalizing to the older human population is immense if age is not included among the variables studied; yet it is common to use pigs that are about four weeks old.

Hannon, J.R., Bossone, C.A. & Wade, C.E. (1990). Normal physiological values for conscious pigs used in biomedical research. Laboratory Animal Science, 40(3).

Subsequent to the derivation of standards of safety based on young animals, the emphasis in applications of the standards is on young people, even though older people are the ones more in danger because they are fragile and often more susceptible. Figuratively speaking, when a public stairway is designed we should try to design it for the people who might have trouble with it, not for the people who would do just as well sliding down a pole.

Investigations of drug interactions are complex because so many factors, so many drugs, so many personal and nutritional variables need to be considered simultaneously. The many additional factors that older people introduce to the problem, with their additional medicines, chronic problems, and special sensitivities, are frequently too much for extant research designs to handle, so these factors are necessarily omitted.

Box 2.6 Research on toxicity

Testing procedures don't accommodate effects of age, as illustrated by the definition of toxic by the Occupational Safety and Health Administration (OSHA): Toxic. A chemical falling within any of the following categories:

1. A chemical that has a median lethal dose (LD-50) of more than 50 milligrams per kilogram but not more than 500 milligrams per kilogram of body weight when administered orally to albino rats weighing between 200 and 300 grams each. (There is no mention of age or sex– and what chemical company in its right financial mind would test for toxicity using a pack of fragile elderly rats?).

2. A chemical that has a median lethal dose (LD-50) of more than 200 milligrams per kilogram but not more than 1,000 milligrams per kilogram of body weight when administered by continuous contact for 24 hours (or less if death occurs within 24 hours) with the bare skin of albino rabbits weighing between two and three kilograms each. (No mention of age.).

3. A chemical that has a median lethal concentration (LC-50) in air of more than 200 parts per million but not more than 2,000 parts per million by volume of gas or vapor, or more than two milligrams per liter but not more than 20 milligrams per liter of mist, fume, or dust, when administered by continuous inhalation for one hour (or less if death occurs within one hour) to albino rats weighing between 200 and 300 grams each.

Throughout there is no mention of age, and it may be that this is a difficult issue to include because of the difference in the aging processes of humans and rats. Certainly the researchers are doing the best they can to serve the general population, but if in fact age of the animals is a significant variable the aged humans are being left out. The use of an animal model such as an albino rat is potentially shaky at the start–is the animal an accurate model of any human? Beyond this, even if the answer is yes, the question arises: Would an elderly albino rat be an adequate model of an older human? This question is very important because of the widespread use of animals in many kinds of testing and requires research.

OSHA (Occupational Safety and Health Administration, US Department of Labor)
Hazard Communication Standards 29 CFR, 1910, 1200.
Website: http://www.osha.gov

For example, older people may be taking MAO (monoamine oxidase) inhibitors, so they must avoid too much red wine and cheese because of the possible inclusion of tyramine. Conversely, young people benefit from such substances because they can assist in dealing with free radicals. On the other hand, older people benefit from some chemicals because they reduce risks of cancer, yet these same chemicals would poison the fetus if a mother were to ingest them. Mathematics exists for sorting out these interactions and for keeping track of all of the biological engines that are humming away inside of us and hopefully appropriate foraging, fomenting and focusing by the mathematical gerontechnologists in collaboration with chemists and biochemists will lead to ways of including older people.

Suggested readings

Birren, J.E. (Ed.). (1996). Encyclopedia of gerontology: Age, aging and the aged. Academic Press, London. ISBN 0-12-226860-1.

Yu, Byung Pal (1993). Free Radicals in Aging. CRC Press, London. ISBN 0-8493-4518-9.

Emerit, I. & Chance, B. (Eds.). (1992). Free radicals and aging. Birkhauser Verlag, Basel. ISBN 0-8176-27448.

Halliwell, B. & Gutteridge, J.M.C. (Eds.). (1998). Free radicals in biology and medicine. 3rd Edition. Oxford University Press, Oxford. ISBN 0-19-850045-9.

Medina, J.J. (1996). The clock of ages: why we age, how we age, winding back the clock. Cambridge University Press, Cambridge. ISBN 0-521-46244-4.

Ricklefs, R.E. & Finch, C.E. (1995). Aging: a natural history. Scientific American Library, Oxford. ISBN 0-7167-5056-2.

Schneider, E.L. & Row, J.W. (Eds.). (1996). Handbook of the biology of aging. 4th Edition. Academic Press, London. ISBN 0-12-627873-3.

Suggested websites

http://www.sfrr.org
Website of the Society for Free Radical Research.

http://www.mayohealth.org/mayo/common/htm
Website of the Mayo Clinic's Health Oasis.

http://www.who.org/ageing
Website of the World Health Organization on Ageing and Health.

http://www.OSHA.gov
Website of OSHA (Occupational Safety and Health Administration.

http://umetech.niwl.se/SCVN/about_ICOH.html
Website of the International Commission on Occupational Health.

CHAPTER THREE

Housing

Introduction

In this chapter we will consider the role of gerontechnology in the area of personal housing, personal as opposed to housing in institutional facilities. Older people may require more specialized houses. This need in turn places specific demands on formulations of housing solutions for the general public because older people are included. "For Rent, No Older people Please," is unacceptable these days. The problem presents a number of interesting opportunities for technology.

In this chapter we will cast about very widely for ideas for technological solutions in housing older people. We will look for ideas in the history of housing of the aging. Similarly, we ask whether useful ideas might come from comparing extremes of culture. Housing in Amsterdam differs from the housing in a Fijian village. Can we borrow ideas in housing from one culture to improve the housing for older people in the other, perhaps even consider "housing" in the animal kingdom? The hope is that we can expand our thinking by sorting through many possible solutions.

First, we define our scope, roughly. With whom are we concerned, and why? What are some of the special characteristics of this population of older people that we need to consider? Gerontechnology subsumes some of sociology. For example, when we do arrive at some technological improvement for a house, how do we distribute it? There are all the social issues of cost, affordability, fairness, and other matters of logistics surrounding this question.

The gerontechnology of housing also subsumes some of psychology. It would be too bad if we were to develop the perfect house and put someone in it only to find that they hated it. So we ask one of the most important questions of all: What kinds of housing do older people in fact want, what nuances? Conversely, what features should we avoid, considering not only those that are dangerous to older people, but also those that are simply inconvenient and annoying to them? A house may be beautifully functional and perfect in almost every way, but how does it feel to the user? Acceptance necessarily involves the psychological complexions of houses. Also, on the psychological plane, how can the older people's desires for housing be fulfilled in ways that do not stigmatize the recipients: for instance, are there ways to simply create solutions that are so good everybody will want to use them, including older people, thus removing the stigma? Overall, there is only one technological question: what does it take to make a house of stones and sticks and bricks and gadgets into a home that protects people and makes them happy?

The scope of gerontechnology in housing

On the one hand, in the area of housing gerontechnology focuses on the healthy older people, most of whom may have needs in housing that overlap completely with those of the general population. In the area of housing, as we see repeatedly in many other contexts, older people can't in any way simply be regarded as a decrepit group that can't climb stairs or turn doorknobs. They don't have scores of debilitating problems that demand complicated houses, which we then devise.

For example, only one percent of individuals over 65 in non-institutional settings use the special equipment for the handicapped in bathrooms (LaPlante et al., 1997). Dementia, of course, changes criteria such as the way-finding requirements that a house must fulfill. Yet survey-based estimates for prevalence of moderate and severe dementia in older populations have ranged from only about 1% to about 14%, centering at around 5%. The percentage of persons needing ramps because they are confined to wheelchairs because of factors related to age is small. And, only few older people experience problems with balance that would require extra railings and extra tactile or visual frames of reference. A number of reviews of the effects of aging exist {Fozard & Heikkinen (1998), Spirduso (1995), Steenbekkers & van Beijsterveldt (1998) and Woollacott & Shumway-Cook (1989)}. The extreme variance shown by the data of Steenbekkers and van Beijsterveldt emphasizes the lack of any clear-cut profile of specific housing needs that we can simply fill.

However, gerontechnology, though dealing with the healthy older people, often has to still take on the full range of disabilities and the needs that may develop associated with them for several reasons.

First, many of the declines that may come with age are gradual and continual and eventually become extreme. They affect everyone including the "healthy," such as the progressive dimming of the light on the retinas by some two-thirds or more at advanced age, which dictates the way houses must be lighted. It is necessary to plan and prepare, of course, as much as possible by providing such features as "level entry" and extra width of the door to accommodate possible future wheel chairs, walkers, shuffling gait and dimmed vision without hindering or endangering people with normal facilities.

Second, designing needs to proceed on a worst-case basis. The house of a fifty-year old needs to be designed with a ninety-year old in mind simply because the tenant will age, or aging parents will move in, or older people will rent or buy the house. The extremes of physical and mental disability toward which older people may eventually drift give us a fairly well defined set of worst-case boundary guidelines for the difficulties that have to be countered. In housing, as in safety, simply planning for the "average" aged person won't work. We have to operate at the extremes as well as near the center. Bouma (1992) cites the "average fallacy" of ergonomics, noting that there is no "average" older person if variations along a number of dimensions are considered. Such a person doesn't exist, so a house built for the average person may well not fit anybody's requirements.

This means that we must think in terms of houses with broadened parameters of design that can help the extremely declined without endangering the normal people, gerontechnology's clients, with a surfeit of contraptions.

Often if we are clever we can expand our scope and encompass the entire range of difficulties by introducing adjustable features into houses, perhaps automatic features, that modify themselves dynamically to accommodate the full range of users when it isn't possible to have one design that fits every separate level of necessity.

Historical examples and sociological perspectives

How have older people been housed in the past? One way was with varieties of group living that appear to have been successful. The "hofjes," units for communal living that were spread throughout the Netherlands and Belgium, can be traced to the middle of the 14th century (Lopes Cardozo, Spruit & Suyderhoud, 1977). Some hofjes have survived the intervening centuries and today, tours are available of such facilities in cities such as Amsterdam and Haarlem. The Bakenesser Kamer in Haarlem has existed since 1395.

The hofjes provided important commonalities. For example there was a common entrance to the square around which the doors of the individual dwellings were situated and this provided a common barrier against the outside world. Common features such as this undoubtedly provided feelings of security. "There is safety in numbers." To harm one member of the group a perpetrator would have to break down "everybody's door" first, a more daunting task.

The church supported some hofjes for poor older people, some were for nuns, and the rich sponsored others: sometimes the hofje was named after the donor in return. These small communities were, formally or not, closed societies. Residents would sit outside and talk together and interact coherently. Many seemed like small villages within the city, for older people. Some were for widows only, some had beautiful reception rooms where the "house lady" of the complex accepted rent each week. The modern extrapolation is the concept of "older leaning," private houses that are in the proximity of an institution for support such as meals and housekeepers.

The equivalent in the United States and elsewhere, for those who can afford it, is the retirement complex where community dining rooms, lounges and classrooms supplement individual dwellings and there are facilities for group transport. Twenty-four hours a day staff is available for emergencies. Some of these communal facilities are now being built on college campuses!

In some sense hofjes shared the principle of "leaning," relying for support on nearby resources. The principle of "Neighborhood Watch" was carried to its logical extreme through the "spy windows" which were large mirrors positioned outside one's window so that it was possible to look directly down the street to see what was going on there, for instance to see when the guests were arriving. The tradition of leaving the curtains open at night exposing the entire living room to all who pass, which is still common in the Netherlands, may be an extension of this thinking–a need for closeness. In the past perhaps the status of the aged was more secure because the social webs were tighter. Still in some countries, but certainly not in countries such as the United States, independent living is less of an issue because older people are taken into the dwellings of their children. Alternately, as it is in some countries of Southern Europe, older people took the children's spouses in when they got married, and also housed their own grandchildren. If the older person lives with the family, there are many benefits, from baby-sitting to keeping the teakettle warmly steaming.

In our modern quest for adequate means of housing older people we in a sense are asking the house to duplicate all of the functions that were, or could possibly have been performed, by people and animals in the past. Sleeping quarters were warmed by the presence of cows, and servants and relatives performed many functions for older people, that we now want the house to perform. Functioning among the people in the colder climates was planned around the stove. Families were tighter. Carrying out activities alone in the remote (cold) regions of the house was less a pleasurable option than it was when central heating became a choice for many near the middle of the 20th century. Now there are trends back toward the stove.

Cultural differences in housing and attitudes toward it

Medical and certain other issues excepted, conceptually at least, in an ideal "primitive" village of long ago, the problems of older people were all solved–because they never existed. Even today, at this moment, in some village in Fiji excited children are jumping around begging to help with the chores of cooking and cleaning in the common kitchen, a structure of grass and wood located centrally among the grass huts in the jungle. These are the same chores that they will take charge of in a few years, and many more years hence their grand children will perform these chores for them.

Box 3.1 Cultural differences in housing

From government to government and from locale to locale, there is extreme variability in sensitivity to the housing needs of older people. In the Netherlands, each citizen of the country is thought to be entitled to a place to live as a basic right of citizenship, complete with a daily newspaper, a phone, transportation to and from the house, and so on. In less favored regions the situation, of course, is much different, as in the countries where many older people simply live in the street.

Needs for housing vary between locations. In some countries people are born on the family boat (boat people) or in the family wagon (gypsies) and never leave it. There exists no need for a house if one has a boat, though some governments have been trying to force these people into apartments and away from their custom of boat dwelling.

Efforts to replace the benefits of village life, piece by piece, are carried out in one way or another in most of the more technologically oriented cultures through a host of channels. Francesco Belletti writes of Vincenza, "Services for older people are provided by various actors: the local municipality (for social problems), health districts (for non-residential health care), private institutions (voluntary groups, non-profit organizations, as well as for-profit companies, managing both residential and home care), and residential facilities."

Leather (1993) cites case studies from other European cities:

Southwest Sector, of Birmingham England, has a "Moving On" service which aims at providing advice and practical support to older home owners needing to move to different houses in order to meet evolving housing and care needs. There are approximately 150 Staying Put, Care and Repair, or similar projects operating throughout Britain. These variously help with affording the cost of building work, repairs, adaptations and improvements, finding a builder, organizing the building work. Birmingham Staying Put is one of 30 projects.

In the Danish case study, one focus is the modernization and adaptation of Pensioners Flats in Copenhagen. Housing is, in some sense, given to older people.

For more than 100 years the goal of the social security and pension systems in Germany has been to insure the economic security of the older person in the phase subsequent to his or her working life.

> If he or she is in need of help, this help is provided according to the subsidiary principle–in the end through the Federal Welfare Act (Bundessozialhilfegesetz–BSHG).
>
> The Dutch case study deals with residential friendly zoning for older people in Amsterdam's district "de Baarsjes."
>
> Among the strategies are:
>
> 1. Providing one central information counter in the district for inhabitants, with information and advice about quality and composition of housing stock, about the new housing projects, waiting times and so on.
> 2. Creation of a fixed number of ordinary dwellings for older people with addition packages of services (designated as "plus dwelling").
> 3. The creation of a network of "neighborhood contact managers."
> 4. The design of a more multicultural society, to smooth out the ethnic group stigmas, yet provide for fraternization within groups.
> 5. Improvement of the existing residential-friendly zones for older people, e.g. improvement of traffic safety and accessibility of the living environment, improvement of social safety, establishing of a meeting place for ethnic groups, improvement of access of dwellings and the creation of plus dwellings.
> 6. Ensuring that dwellings suitable to older people are reserved for older people only.

So it is with the other tasks that support the village and its people, older people included. As soon as you are old enough, you work helping to build the wall of rocks around the village to keep out the river at high tide, or you work in town, or weave baskets, or fish. And when you are too old you gradually retire from these tasks and they are performed for you just as you have been performing them for your own parents. Simply being a member of the village is its own investment plan–you invest your time. Your retirement plan is simple, "Retire from whichever activities you care to, whenever you feel like it, with unrestricted options to 'un-retire' tomorrow, permanently or just for the afternoon." You are never lonely because you are never alone. You have whatever amount of contact with your fellow seniors, life-long friends, or relatives, you may desire. Your children are all around you, with their own children.

You have respect–because you are old, and experienced; you know the old stories, the triumphs and defeats of the village long since past, you know how to make the village work and you know how to relate to the jungle. When you become even older and begin to forget these things–it doesn't really matter. Ironically, many of our modern problems in the gerontechnology of housing can be captured in only one question: how do we give our older people all of the physical, psychological and social luxuries of a simple hut in a good village?

The answer depends on the specific cultural context in which the question is asked. Let's take a look at a few representative efforts here and there. One remedy, bristling with cultural dimensions, is "kangaroo housing" where children add on an extra room to the house to serve as a pouch in which the older parents can ride. It is cultural in terms of its degree of acceptance by both children and parents. Both the youth and older people of some cultures seem attracted to this closeness, some others favor it less highly or hold it in negative regard. In the south of Europe older people tend to live with their children more than do seniors in the North. In other countries a dozen people or more may sleep in one room, and then the entire conception of privacy is nonexistent and there is no need even for a separate pouch for parents.

At least one construction company actually specializes in such additions. Building part of a house has advantages. If the unit is to be newly built it can be built correctly so that it conforms not only to the requirements of older people, but also to these specific seniors. And building part of a house that can simply be plugged in to the main house's power and other facilities is certainly less costly than building an entire house.

The distribution of appropriate housing

Finding ways to distribute proper housing fairly is a major problem. Satisfying needs, even though the technology may exist, is an exercise in design, logistics, and distribution. For one thing, old people don't tend to live in new houses. Some solutions can only be incorporated in housing stock that is newer and beyond the financial grasp of many older people. So a large group may be out of phase with the technology that is supposed to help them. This factor presses us to provide solutions that are not only cheap, but also relatively portable so that everyone can benefit. Built-in features for older people are appealing in some ways, but may be unattainable within appropriate time frames. Ideally, shortly after the piece of technology is produced it should be implementable cheaply and to the extent desired, and be tailored to older people. Thus a part of gerontechnology involves leveraging industry to incorporate older people in its designs, decisions, and schemes for marketing and distribution.

This issue of mechanisms of social support for housing is very deserving of the consideration of gerontechnologists because it dramatically affects older people. Perhaps as important, it plagues the thinking of the young as well. In countries where there is no guaranteed support, there is a subtle life-long preoccupation–"What am I going to do when..."

Some representative problems with typical housing

Safety from accidents

Perhaps the most pressing problems involve safety and the necessity for older people to constantly be worrying about it. Employing mental simulation to gain insight, imagine that you have become extremely old. A friend has dropped you off at the sidewalk in front of your house. You shuffle slowly toward the mailbox by the curb. You know that the metal handle is sharp, the hinges are corroded, your hands are weak and the slightest exertion of force makes the joints hurt: you know that the pain will remain for hours after the force is gone. "Is it worth it? No, nobody writes; maybe I'll wait and check the mail tomorrow." You slowly proceed down the sidewalk. Keep your feet apart as you walk for safety even though you may not be able to lift them high above the cement and they scrape along. A fall to either side could break your hip, it happened to your friend. Look down, always down. A one-centimeter rise in the cement will trip a person who shuffles, and you get preoccupied in thought you know. Look very carefully because the sidewalk is just a blur. You might not notice the crack until too late. Finally, here come the four steps to the porch. Slow up! If you go too fast, stiffness in the knees may prevent your foot from clearing the lip of a step.

Box 3.2 Senior label for housing

In the Netherlands a system for rating houses in terms of their suitability for older people exists. It is called "Seniorenlabel" or Senior label. This system was created in 1993 as an experimental certificate of consumer quality in housing. The requirements are broken into the environment, the building and the home:

The environment:
Public transport within walking distance (500 m).
Shops for daily provisions and post office/bank easily reached
  (500m of walking, perhaps to public transport).
Good access routes from the public highway to the home/building.
Sufficient lighting in the immediate vicinity of the home (including on paths
  and in car parks).

The building:
Sufficient lighting in and around the building (100 lux at 1 meter).
All entrance accessories accessible and usable by everyone.
Minimal height differences at thresholds (at maximum 2 cm).
Sufficiently large doors (at least 1.05 m).
Sufficient space around doors (2 x 2 m).
A lift suitable for wheelchair users.
Safe stair and stairrails (height 85-95 cm, diameter 3-5 cm).
Sufficiently wide halls and galleries.

The home:
All primary rooms at the same level or accessible by safe stairs.
Safe stair rails (height 85-95 cm, diameter 3-5 cm).
No thresholds inside.
Sufficiently large doors (at least 1.05 m).
Sufficient space around doors (2 x 2 m).
Secure door hardware.
Operation of windows, doors and electric switches is safe, practicable
  and accessible to everyone.
Three room home.
Lighting by each outside door (100 lux at 1 meter).
All entrance accessories accessible and usable by everyone.
Adequate space for furniture.
Large enough kitchen and bedrooms.
A safe shower.
Toilet is accessible for wheelchair users.
Bathroom is suitable (or can be made suitable) for users of wheel chairs.
Access to outdoor area (balcony, terrace).
Fitted with a central heating system of sufficient capacity.

http://www.seniorenlabel.nl

And, because you're reacting much too slowly to recover from a trip these days, you'll certainly fall and probably something will break. You're like an eggshell and you know it. But if you go slowly up the steps it means balancing on one foot at a time, precariously. With an aging sense of balance your world doesn't hold as still as it used to, the stair underfoot doesn't feel level even when it is either. Your sense of self-motion is often wrong. You can't hold the railing they put on for you because you're carrying your groceries.

We leave you to proceed in this inside the house, put everything away, cook supper, clean up, take a shower in a slippery bathtub, and go to bed. Good luck!

It's true this is an outlandish description of aging that simply doesn't apply in most cases, but as we noted, we need to design for the extremes. If the environment can't hurt the decrepit it won't hurt the normal people either, even when they may be acting decrepit for whatever reason. It doesn't hurt to grind down the breaks in the sidewalk–no one will trip on them if you do, someone eventually will if you don't. It doesn't hurt to fix all of these things–design and maintain as though in fact you were doing it for the person in the example–think and design the house for the worst case even though this case doesn't really exist in the form of one single person.

Part of the things that are wrong with the typical normally safe and convenient houses in terms of safe accessibility are obvious. They can be detected easily with a simple mental "walk-through," such as this. Others are obscure, totally obscure. Let's unmask a couple of hidden hazards to illustrate.

The average house is subtly booby trapped for the aged

Some hidden hazards are difficult to detect and while some don't actually cause problems, they set the resident up for situations involving multiple converging factors that cause the person to react inappropriately–the person causes the problem. These hazards are hidden, not in space but in time, in sequences of events.

For example, a cold bathtub or bathroom floor can be very dangerous just because it's cold. Why? Shouldn't the coefficients of friction even be greater then? Here's why: The sensory receptors that signal cold to the brain are distributed more in the arch side of the skin of the foot than along the outer part–it is very unpleasant when the arch of your foot touches a cold floor. Without realizing it, some people, maybe all walk on the outside edges of the feet to avoid that unpleasant feeling. This is a very unstable way to walk because it deprives us of a standard recovery maneuver. One way humans avoid tipping over to the outside (one of the most dangerous kinds of fall) is by rolling the ankle outward. This moves the center of support, now the edge of the foot, quickly outward and more underneath the person. Walking with the ankle already rolled outward deprives one of this maneuver. It also lowers the coefficients of friction because this part of the foot doesn't grip the floor as well. These factors predispose one to a slip and fall to the outside.

If the floor were merely cold there might be a problem, but, to make things much worse, people also reflexively tend to walk this way if the floor is wet, to keep their feet partially dry after toweling them. Then, in addition, the floor is slippery and one probably shouldn't be walking on it even flat-footed.

Post-traumatic amnesia–why we may not learn about problems in our houses

Why don't we learn not to do this after a few close-call slips and maybe a fall or two? First, because we don't even realize that we do such things. Scientific investigators aren't commonly allowed to observe unstructured bathroom behavior. And second, because if there is a close call or a fall, then retrograde amnesia sets in. People can have trouble remembering what happened immediately before a disaster, so they can't learn from the accident.

As an aside, this illustrates that the gerontechnologist can sometimes profit by being a generalist. The obvious problems in the lives of older people can simply be listed and corrected. The complicated problems in a house, such as the one above require a great deal more analysis. Pause for a moment to consider what was involved in identifying and formulating the foregoing case of the cold tile floor. We needed to think about distributions of sensory nerves, the cold receptors. This is sensory neurophysiology. We had to consider coefficients of friction on different parts of the skin and gripping power of the foot in different configurations, that is, the biomechanics of the foot, which involves physics. We needed behavioral analysis to understand how people walk. We needed to know about amnesia of human memory and assorted other things.

Sensory systems of houses: Instrumenting the house for chemical awareness

Houses are subject to contamination, radon, smoke, subtle poisons, fumes, and allergens. But humans aren't very good at smelling poison in the first place, and the sense of smell may decline with age. Many clever techniques exist that can be modified and applied to monitor the environments of older people. Consider some sources of ideas. Food scientists use "tasters" to make sure that food is safe, for instance, mice that are fed shellfish to test for poison. Similarly, royalty of the past sometimes had other people taste their food to test it for poison. Today, the technology of chemical "sniffers" is growing rapidly. Just as truffle growers can use truffle pigs that can smell truffles under the ground and the food and wine industries employ professional human sniffers and tasters for detecting and identifying contaminants, houses can be olfactorily endowed.

For example, reminiscent of the dogs that sniff for explosives and drugs at the airport, in the microscopic domain of our world, "molecule dogs" are used to sniff out specific molecules, with extreme sensitivity. These are bacteria whose cell membranes can't develop in the presence of specific substances such as penicillin. This alerts the scientist to the presence of the molecule.

Of course, this suggests a novel source for the technology of protection, animal trainers and the pet industry. They could train personal molecule hounds for the houses of older people in the form of small birds, insects, microbes and mammals that don't tolerate pollutants as well as people do or that can recognize them and signal.

Box 3.3 Domotics

Without the nervous system to take in sensory information, coordinate movement and a hundred other things, humans and other living creatures would be in dire straits. Presently, most houses are in just this condition. They have a few primitive senses, such as for room temperature, and a few primitive cognitive/motor links to these, such as the thermostat that decides when the room is too cold or too hot and turns the furnace on or off. But the thermostat usually doesn't know about even simple things such as the time of day or about the calendar. Still, some thermostats do know that the furnace shouldn't run all night, that people sleep in on weekends, and a few other helpful, if trivial things. But they don't usually know what rooms, which people are in, or their individual preferences for temperature. They don't have remote controls let alone respond to spoken commands of the user.

Domotics involves the communication between electronic and other devices in their interaction with the user. It is especially important for older people in terms of comfort, for heat and humidity, filtering of dust, and in terms of safety with burglar alarms, shower temperatures, and other sorts of awarenesses and concerns that the house can offer the user. In addition, there are the goals of convenience, comfort, communication, the delivery of information, and entertainment.

As the computerization of houses gains ground it will become easier and easier to add features because much of the hardware will already be in place and standardized. For example, the BUS (Binary Unit System) allows a variety of devices to communicate. And when a new device needs to be added it is simply plugged in on the bus. Instantly it is physically "wired" to all of the other instruments. It becomes functionally connected also, if the appropriate software is in place. Outfitting the house for features and flexibility is taking the same direction that the manufacture of automobiles has gone. It is best to install all of the electro/optical and computer facilities for all of the features that may be eventually needed. Then if the user wants to have a new feature, perhaps have the curtains automatically drawn closed when the house senses someone outside the house or pulled open ten minutes after the toaster comes on in the morning, it's just a matter of programming.

http://www.batibus.com
Website for "on-line" buildings.

http://www.ehsa.com
Website of the European Home Bus Association.

But, synthetic technological "pets" may soon do as well. For instance, one enzyme molecule can lead to the production of thousands or millions of target molecules, and these can then easily be detected and analyzed. Fluidizing beds can be used in the detection of a few molecules of chemical, and methods of amplifying samples of DNA now reach similar levels of relative sensitivity. These provide extreme leverage from technology that is available now and that lets us approach the single molecule level in analyzing the environments of older people for hazards.

Safety from molecules and particles in the house involves a very complicated tangle of interacting factors, aspects of the house, of the individual person, interactions with the weather, humidity, and so on. Many people are working on these problems as they affect seniors.

A number of studies worldwide are being carried out on the indoor environment, not just in relation to sensing pollutants, but also in conjunction with a number of the other issues. For example, a significant percentage of older people have compromised pulmonary functioning–their lungs not only fail to extract oxygen from the air as well as they once did, they also become hyper-reactive to specific substances that are found in the atmosphere of the house. They can sense some of these themselves, such as dust. One can see dust and feel its effects in the nose. But other pollutants, such as debris from house mites require the special sensors.

The spatial distributions of pollutants such as house mites and their effects, once known, can provide foundations for developing special techniques of housekeeping, as well as techniques for synchronizing factors such as humidity and ventilation to optimize the quality of the air in the house.

Some dimensions of aging as they bear on adequacy of housing

Physical ability

According to a National Center for Health Statistics Advance Data survey (Kovar & La Croix, 1987), the following difficulties with motion prevail. About eleven percent of people in their fifties have difficulty walking up ten steps. Twenty-one percent of people of age 70-74 have difficulty, and about nine percent can't do it at all. Around twenty percent of people in their fifty's have trouble stooping, crouching, or kneeling. By ages 70-74 the percentage has risen to about 38 percent and seventeen percent of this age group cannot perform the action at all. The percentage for ages between 70 and 74 who can't reach up overhead, about eight; who can't grasp things, about six percent; who can't lift or carry a 12 kilogram weight, around nine percent. This is a survey of workers. Many people with severe difficulties disqualify themselves from working of course. But this group appears to get along very well and most of them wouldn't be expected to have much trouble in an average house. There have been hundreds of attempts at measuring the capacities of the old in general, by self-report and a host of objective measures. For our purposes the message in housing that comes from these is "customization." Most of older people don't share a common set of problems that just get worse and worse with age. The problems are idiosyncratic so the houses must also be. Of course, we make all of the doors easy to open, all of the floors difficult to fall on, and so forth. But when a person has problems it is likely that they will be uniquely peculiar to that person and the house will have to respond in a unique way. Nevertheless, some efforts at standardization are quite helpful. In the Netherlands a Senior label has been developed.

The house's memory and task orientation

NASA and other agencies concerned with the quality of performance break the tasks down in terms of "work load"–who does what, and who decides? So it is with an older person in a house: what does the person do; what does the house do? To illustrate the point, imagine that some person is prone to mental preoccupation, forgetting parts of some routines, neglecting to turn off the burner of the stove, leaving the water running or the door unlocked, or the window open.

Protection of the resident who may do these things from time to time can proceed along two lines. The functions can be performed automatically by the house so that failing to perform them doesn't make any difference–the house can do it all, just as an airliner can almost land itself; or the house can generate signals, mental prompts and other coaching with respect to tasks it can't or isn't allowed to handle, or the house and the person can negotiate, or the house can just sit there and be only a simple house, with no domotics.

To get some feel for the technicalities that are involved, think about designing a system that guarantees that the doors are never left unlocked, but one that doesn't ever lock the door with the resident standing outside with no key, that doesn't frustrate the resident, that is wary of criminals and can't be tricked by them, and that deals with animals and children.

Orientation and guidance of locomotion

At the extreme, an older person may tend to forget where things are, or forget how to do things or how to move about the house, in which case the house can remind, or obviate the need for remembering. The house should implicitly explain its own layout so that not only the older resident, but perhaps first-time visitors as well, can know how to get to the bathroom, or go outside, especially in the case of an emergency.

Way finding and orienting one's self take on new dimensions at night where older people are concerned. Walking to the bathroom, or escaping the premises require clear perceptual aides that can be seen even with the lowered sensitivity to visual contrast that the older people may have. For example, glowing guidelines or blinking beacons can be devised. Of course, the increased sensitivity to glare of the older person can render him or her virtually blind under conditions of low illumination if a light source that is intended to guide people is shining into the eyes. Auditory beacons can be dangerous because the ability to localize sounds often fails in older people. Perhaps in the worst case, sounds may be perceived as coming from incorrect directions, "guiding" the person incorrectly.

Box 3.4 Home bus standardization

To exchange information between appliances a bus system is required. Technologically speaking various systems are possible depending on requirements and costs, but only the universal adoption of a single standard will lead to mass production of components and low prices.

In the mid-eighties the European Commission (EC) received proposals to support experiments with particular bus systems. It soon became clear that the various groups were coming up with different bus systems. The wild growth of bus systems was undesirable as it made potential users to adopt an attitude of waiting. In order to correct the situation initiative was taken to set up a European Home Bus Association with the mission arriving at a unified bus system in Europe. The idea was that the EC should only support projects that would be in line with that mission. It also became clear that the market was not developing as quickly as was initially anticipated. This made companies less eager to invest.

This situation forced the market leaders in building automation to make a decisive step to come to a convergence of European bus systems. This new international body endorses standardized data communication in building automation with a completely flexible structure–a prerequisite for almost unlimited configurability, compatibility with all areas of building automation and easy integration of external functions. Based on the electrical network installation, the new standard combines the best features of the existing bus systems BatiBUS, EHS, and EIB, and concerns itself on a world-wide basis with all aspects of building automation whether in residential housing or commercial and industrial buildings. Ultimo 1999 it led to a new organization in Brussels, The Universal Bus Association, TUBA, which centralizes all standardizing activities of the member founders. Representatives of the various companies now work in the same group and in the same building. Finally the original idea of one European standard in building automation has become close.

Beside the European standard there are other bus systems in the world. In the USA there is a virtual standard, as well as in Japan. These standards differ from the European one, and even worse, they are not compatible.

http://www.batibus.com
Website for "on-line" buildings.

http://www.ehsa.com
Website of the European Home Bus Association.

Safe ambulation in the dark at night demands that the floor be uncluttered: because the older person may have less facility for recovering balance if there is a trip, and because the consequences of a fall can be much higher. Thus, if the older person hasn't the energy, the inclination, or the ability to put things away, the house must provide judiciously designed and placed storage for items that might otherwise be put on the floor, such as convenient hangers, drawers, and hooks. In the case of some items, such as dirty laundry, throw-bins can be provided.

The technology exists to allow the house to be endowed with some cleverness about warning of objects on the floor that might trip the older person. As with the radar in a control tower at an airport, a dimmed laser beam could be swept a fraction of an inch above the carpet to create an invisible sheet of light above the footing of the passageway that would reflect from any objects left in the path and would light the footing ahead by bouncing off the slippers and onto the floor. Or slippers could be equipped with LED headlights, or the house could simply turn on its lights, at a low level to prevent flash blindness to which older people are more vulnerable, when it sensed someone moving.

Visual information in the house

As visual acuity and sensitivity to contrast decline with aging, the labels on stoves, thermostats, dish washers, washing machines, dryers, radios, and other items need to be larger, to be free from glare, and need to contrast more strongly than usual with their backgrounds. The house can be designed or retrofitted so that such labels are readable, or sensory substitutions can be devised. The burners of the stove can be marked with highly visible color codes and the control buttons can be individually colored accordingly so that normal reading isn't even necessary. The house can alleviate some sensory deficits of age: magnifying glasses can hang by the medicine cabinet or in other locations where acuity might be a problem.

Box 3.5 Domestic hazards

Older people tend to spend more time at home than younger adults. The typical house, however, in a sense is sometimes a minefield of potential danger. About half of all accidents occur in or around the home. Older people may well be more vulnerable to certain mishaps or accidents. Insight is needed to foresee the problems and take preventive action.

Let us consider the complexities of a few of the hazards in one small region, the bathroom.

Footing. Friction needs be neither too low nor too high. A low friction may lead to slipping and falling backward, a high friction to scuffing and falling forward. It may be safer to err in the direction of too much friction, because a forward fall may be less dangerous than a backward fall. The optimal friction depends on whether the person wears shoes, slippers, or just goes barefoot. In the bathroom, the friction may change unexpectedly because of a wet surface or spilled soap or shampoo. Small carpets outside or within the shower area may unexpectedly slip. Solutions can be found in developing and applying safer materials, in specific designs in which wet or soapy spots are less likely, in providing handrails and other supports, and in a heightened awareness of the hazards by proper education of the users.

Escalating sequences of events. Falls may occur as the end products of chains of events that develop over the course of a few seconds. For example, the user may misstep slightly, leading to a recovery maneuver such as a quick step sideward to reestablish balance. There may be something in the way, which calls for a new recovery maneuver. This may lead an older person, perhaps already endowed with some unsteadiness, to fall. Other triggering events may be inadvertently touching hot pipes or reaching out too high up or too far away to some soap dish or to the temperature adjustment, or to the light switch or to the power socket for the hair dryer.

Other hazards may include cupboards that are too high, in combination with temptations to climb on anything available such as an unsteady stool or chair. The safety of the bathroom therefore requires a careful ergonomic design taking into account any special habits of the users. For persons specifically vulnerable to falls, such as in cases of osteoporosis, other preventive measures may be considered or developed as well, such as wearing protective clothing or even little airbags.

Levón, B-V. & Kaakinen, J. (1998). Safety for the elderly by improving the environment. In: Graafmans, J., Taipale, V., and Charness, N. (Eds.). Gerontechnology. A sustainable investment in the future. IOS Press, Amsterdam. ISBN 90-5199-367-6.

Perceptual and cognitive dimensions

There are hundreds and hundreds of dimensions of personal capability that are important when we think about designing houses. Some of these have been worked out with respect to the aged, most haven't. Let us illustrate here by considering the narrowing of the visual field. What are the consequences? Loss of vision, or loss of awareness of the periphery make people more susceptible to knocking things over, tripping, and failing to see information. To appreciate the situation more fully, get the tube from an empty role of paper towels and make a sandwich while looking only through it. This simulation is extreme of course; few people are quite so debilitated. But it conveys the general problem well. What would you add to a standard kitchen in the area where sandwiches are made to offset such a loss?

On the cognitive side of making this sandwich, some older people need to perform tasks more serially as they age if they have trouble doing several things at once. However, as you no doubt noticed when you were seeing the world serially one small glimpse at a time through your paper tube, it takes longer to do things serially. You have to look for the butter, and only after you find it can you look for the tomatoes, and when you find them maybe you've forgotten where the butter was. Life is much easier when you see a complete visual field. If you don't have one, the house needs to be arranged to accommodate for your serial performance.

Examples of innovative technical solutions and systems

Several countries have installed model houses, demonstrating in tangible reality how a house for seniors might look and providing a testing ground for new ideas. Intelligent houses are developed in a field known as "Domotics." A model house is an excellent advertisement for the cause of gerontechnology.
Among the features of a smart house are counter tops that can be adjusted for wheel chair accessibility, switches and levers that are easy to manipulate, computerized security systems, safe bathing facilities with grips and seats. Additional forms of technology could be incorporated such as special equipment to assist caregivers with lifting, and pressure sensitive

beds and floors to provide early warning of falls. In Finland the Marjala project similarly exhibits solutions for older people.

The first house that might have assisted older people, the first smart house, was shown in the New York world's fair in 1939 (Blaich, 1992).
Today, many "smart house" devices, which are applicable to older people, have already been offered to the public. For example, there are companies that integrate and regulate security systems, lighting, heating and cooling, entertainment systems, and many convenience options. These systems can control automatic blinds and drapes, gas and electric fireplaces, security cameras, electronic locks, major appliances, and more.

Crestron Remote Control Systems provides a convenient interface with such systems, using commonly meaningful pictures and words on a touch screen to provide a remote control system that is literally at the fingertips. You see a floor plan of your house, touch the room of your choice, and the lights are adjusted or the temperature controlled, or you can control your home's music and video. Or you can manipulate doors and gates, deal with pools and spas or with your satellite systems and other appliances.

JDS Technologies of San Diego, CA, offers a method of controlling your house by telephone, locally or from a distant location, among other things, and allows a number of functions to be timed such as assistive switching devices, motion detectors using X-10 (a standardized controller language that can be used to send control signals over the house's power wiring), infrared, and devices that are hard-wired.
Several magazines are presently dedicated to the discussion of such devices, for example Popular Home Automation and The Electronic House, and there are countless technological projects in the magazines for electronic hobbyists that apply to the problems of older people.

Next, because our purpose is to stimulate the reader's thoughts and actions for the future, rather than dwell too much on the achievements of the past, we turn to a few developments that are on the way, and follow with some successes that ought to become available someday, if the gerontechnologists can find ways to arrive at them.

As might be expected, there are many available modules and systems that would allow an older person to control the house and its appliances by voice commands. At the Media Laboratory of the Massachusetts Institute of Technology, Pentland's group is attempting to move considerably beyond even that. Pentland notes that contemporary computers are usually both deaf and blind. So the group has developed a family of computer systems for recognizing faces, expression, and gestures. The system will know who is in the room and where they are, will know things about the person such as preferences and tendencies, will be able to see emotions on the faces and will react appropriately to what the people are doing, saying, gesturing about, or feeling.

The smart what?

In gerontechnology we have to stretch our thinking beyond normal limits until your mind says; "Wait a minute, this is going too far! It's technically impossible to develop this particular feature; this feature would get in the way; this level of analysis of daily life is too detailed and intrusive!" Then pause and try to devise a way to answer your own objection, realizing that you are thinking for a world 50 years in the future, not necessarily for present society. For example, the very idea of some inquisitive toilet knowing who you are, knowing what your personal parameters are and your medical data, is unsettling: devise and incorporate optional anonymity without sacrificing data. Think flexibly. It may not be possible for a wonder refrigerator to measure thyroid levels, so measure correlated variables such as the dynamics of muscle tension.

Box 3.6 Smart toilet

The toilet may be a place of private difficulties. Can technology help to make the toilet a better place?

Consider features that have recently been developed to make toilet use easier for everybody but certainly for people who have difficulty moving the legs, body or arms, for example as may stem from rheumatism. Difficulties in mobility are among the most frequent functional disorders of older people. A compatible toilet then is height adjustable and, as a matter of course, has supports to make sitting down and standing up easier. It has a warm water nozzle for easy cleaning such as in a French bidet and a warm air stream for quick drying. Do not think that these features are sheer luxury. If we take into account the difficulties and effort required in regular toilets without such features, and in particular the professional or informal help that many frail people need for their toilet use, including the embarrassment involved and the involuntary waiting times, there may well be large returns on the necessary investment. This is particularly true for nursing homes. In fact, a recently built nursing home connected to the National Institute for Longevity Studies in Nagoya, Japan, has installed only toilets that include most of the above comforts.

Now let us take the issue a step further. The smart toilet (Personal communication, Herbig, 1996) has much added functionality and can monitor a number of physiological variables that are indicative of the momentary state of health. The smart toilet detects who you are, measures your weight before and after toilet use, watches for dehydration and analyses excretions for a number of substances and checks for normal or deviating values. On the basis of the analyses, it advises you to drink somewhat more or much more. If necessary it assembles information about medicine use, blood sugar, tests for internal bleeding, always taking into account both general norms and individual past profiles. It will know if your diet is remaining effective and will make suggestions for types and levels of food intake and exercise. It may deliver a print out, and send deviating results to your doctor's computer.
The smart toilet is not yet here but the concept seems promising in particular for regulation of medication and diet and prevention of disease. The feedback to the user should be carefully filtered in order to not create too high a level of continuous concern, nor be too technical. Recommendations or instructions that might appeal to a computer model may not be appropriate in instructing the person on how to regulate parameters of one's normal varying lifestyle.

Tamura, T., Togawa, T., Ogawa, M. & Yamakoshi, K. (1998) Fully Automated Health Monitoring at Home. In: Graafmans, J., Taipale, V. & Charness, N. (Eds.). (1998). Gerontechnology A sustainable investment in the future. Proceedings of the second International Conference on Gerontechnology, Helsinki, October 1996.
IOS Press, Amsterdam. ISBN 90-5199-367-6.

Bear in mind of course that any device, psychologically speaking could either provide one of the worst, or one of the best experiences on the planet for older people: nobody knows yet. Experimentation after development and application of technology is always required to see whether the new offering is really manageable and really appreciated. Marketing to seniors is as perfidious as the rest of marketing. No market researcher would have predicted that anyone in his right mind would ever actually be able to, or would dare to, hurdle along at 20 km/h sitting on a 15 cm seat balanced precariously on only two wheels, while simultaneously flailing the feet about in circular orbits–dare to ride a bicycle.

Suggested readings

Brink, S. (Ed.). (1998). Housing older people: an international perspective. Transaction Publishers, London. ISBN 0-7658-0416-6.

Golant, S.M. (1992). Housing America's elderly. Sage publications, Newbury Park, CA, USA. ISBN 0-8039-4763-X.

Habraken, N.J. (1970). Three R's for Housing. Scheltema & Holkema, Amsterdam. ISBN 90-6060-014-2.

Russell, L. (1999). Housing options for older people. Age Concern, London. ISBN 0-8624-2287-6.

Steenbekkers, L.P.A. & Beijsterveldt, C.E.M. van (Eds.). (1998). Design-relevant characteristics of ageing users: Backgrounds and guidelines for product innovation. Delft University Press, Delft. ISBN 90-407-1709-5.

Suggested websites

http://www.smart-homes.nl
Website of the Foundation Smart Homes.

http://www.caba.org
Website of the Continental Automated Buildings Association, North America's key source for information, education, and networking relating to home and building automation.

http://www.adaptenv.org/aboutaec.htm
Website of the Adaptive Environments Center.

CHAPTER FOUR

Lifelong Working

Introduction

In this chapter, first we will examine some of the problems that exist, both for older people in the workplace and for older people who have stopped working. These are related to a number of complex factors that involve a person's changing levels of competence with age balanced against the changing demands for competence of the modern workplace, and against the psychological factors such as feelings of self worth and loneliness. In retirement, there may be too much spare time, and a decline of personal finances. On the social side, there are pressures on governments and companies to conserve money while increasing productivity.

We are expecting a swell of older workers in the future

There is some urgency. Issues in employment are always modulated by the ever-changing blend of ages within a society. We all know that there are more older individuals working now. The baby boomers, born after the Second World War, reached late middle age at the end of the nineties; meanwhile there was a lower birth rate in the Western World between 1975 and 1995. Older people gained numbers in the workplace while the number of young diminished. In the late 1990's the most strongly represented age group was between 40 and 50. In 2010, Ilmarinen (1996) predicts that many commercial firms will find their largest proportion of workers to be between 55 and 65. In the past, many adults worked to support only a few old people. The average life span 2000 years ago was perhaps in the teens or twenties. Given the explosion in technology, we may soon exceed that figure by a factor of 5 or more and governments have to plan accordingly for a day when almost everyone is old and nearly no one is young. According to a study of the WHO, in 2020 the average age in Europe will be near 60. Who are these older workers? What are they really like?

In what sense do people decline at work?

Do they?

Certainly, sometimes it may be true that when people try to stay on the same jobs into old age, the workplace may start to outdistance their changing profiles of personal ability, technologically in terms of performance or production. The assembly line moves too quickly, the hammer is too heavy, and the printing on the gauge or the page is too small. However, performance obviously depends on many factors such as the type of work that is involved and the characteristics of the individual.
In strenuous activities such as mining the main issue is strength, which declines. Although one small slight man of 104 years educated everyone in this regard by lifting a man of over 90 kg, Ed McMahon, on a television show one night, that isn't what one commonly sees.
There is a balance between the dimensions of the task and the dimensions of the worker. In watch making and neurosurgery the currency is steadiness, which can go either way, improve or diminish. In musicianship, hearing is important but it may decline along some dimensions with age as it improves along others. The highly varying demands of tasks underscores the near impossibility of treating older people in the workplace as any sort of homogeneous stereotypical group requiring any consistent adjustments.

Some facets of our involvement

In 1991, a Study Group of the World Health Organization (WHO) on Aging and Working Capacity convened. The need for this meeting and the nature of the objectives exemplify the various roles of gerontechnology in the area of aging and work. These individual objectives of the WHO are presented below, paired with the corresponding roles of gerontechnology to illustrate our intended coverage in the area of working.

Box 4.1 Work ability index

Many nations have been interested in assessing and predicting the future capabilities of aging workers. The Finnish Institute of Health (Ilmarinen & Tuomi, 1993) developed the Work ability index in the 80's. This questionnaire can be used in periodic occupational health examinations. Work ability is expressed as a discrete figure, ranging from 7 - 49.

	Scale
1. Work ability now related to life's best level	0 -10
2. Work ability related to work demands Physical work and Mental work	2 -10
3. Number of chronic diseases	1 - 7
4. Handicap due to the disease	1 - 6
5. Absence due to sickness	1 - 5
6. Prognosis for the next 2 years	1 - 7
7. Mental resources	1 - 4
Range	7 -49

Poor work ability= 7-27, moderate = 28-43, good = 44-49.

There are undesirable factors in the workplace that should be avoided:

Excessive physical demands. In this category are: Static muscular work; use of muscular strength; lifting and carrying; sudden extreme effort; repetitive movements; simultaneously bent and twisted work postures.

Stressful and dangerous work environment. These items include: Dirty and wet workplaces; risk of work accidents; hot workplaces; cold workplaces; changes in temperature during the working day; poor lighting.

Poor organization of work. The most important issues were deemed to be: Conflicts of responsibilities; unsatisfactory supervision and planning of work; fear of failure and mistakes; time pressures; lack of freedom of choice; lack of control over one's own work; lack of professional development; lack of acknowledgement and appreciation.

Ilmarinen stresses that work ability is an interaction between the individual's physical, mental, and social skills and the demands of the workplace. Decreased work ability will result from decreased recognition at work, deteriorating tools, and increased standing in the work setting as well as lessened exercise during leisure activities. He also concludes that it isn't enough to just keep on working. Active steps must be taken to maintain the ability to work.

Ilmarinen, J. & Tuomi, K. (1993). Workability index for aging workers. In: J. Ilmarinen. (Ed.). Aging and work 2. (pp. 142-151). FIOH, Helsinki. ISBN 951-801-915-0.

The WHO objectives:

1. To analyze changes in work capacity due to aging in relation to employment policy and sustained development in all member states.
   A typical role of gerontechnology is in searching for or stimulating new developments in computerized modeling and mathematical analysis that can be used in describing and assessing the worker in the workspace in relation to the dynamic changes in work capacity of the worker.
   The objective is to balance ability and demand. For example, much of the work on task analysis, workload, analysis of work spaces, control dynamics, or tool design, such as that done by NASA, by TNO Institute of Human Factors in Soesterberg, the Netherlands, and by similar groups, is appropriate for modeling. The resulting models, in turn, can be related to policy models.

2. To study the biological background of aging, leading to changes in physical and mental capacity for adapting to work requirements.
   Much of the substance of gerontechnology comes from fields such as biochemistry, physiology, physiological psychology, and the psychology of stress as they apply to aging and to its implications for performance.

3. To identify health problems related to changes in work capacity among the aging workforce. Gerontechnology is in league with medical science as a source of methods for assessing dimensions of health that might underlie problems on the job. Of particular importance is occupational health care–screening for problems at the workplace. Is the lighting too dim? Is the table too high? Is the noise level potentially injurious?

4. To define areas for health promotion in aging working populations. Gerontechnology, in its Preventive and Enhancement modes, is allied with pertinent fields such as ergonomics and biomechanics, that are important in the analysis and maintenance of physical performance to avert problems such as repetitive strain injuries or injuries from lifting.

5. To define a strategy and develop recommendations to help member states to overcome the health problems related to aging working populations and the changes in their work capacity. One arm of gerontechnology focuses on proselytizing and advertising the causes of older people, raising awareness and teaching new attitudes, in order to expose the problems of older people at work to the relevant political entities.

6. To identify gaps in knowledge and areas for further research. The gerontechnologist is first an analyst, in collaboration with the older workers themselves, mapping both the findings and shortcomings of modern technology onto the terrain with which older people must deal in the workplace.

These then are the important issues, but all in a sense related to decline rather than compatibility: the WHO seems to have no concern if there is general pathological decline.
WHO in these statements gives no attention to the more positive outlook and approaches, for instance, training in situ, and support of information/communication.

The vocabulary of "decline"

However, instead of focusing so much always on degradation, perhaps a clearer conception of older people's situation, for gerontechnology at least to grapple with, would be to focus more on compatibility of the person and the job. Often a few relatively minor details can be adjusted here and there, rather than turning to something drastic such as reassignment or retirement. This approach requires attention to the specifics as opposed to the generalities.

The WHO Study Group concurs in their phrasing with many who have done research on aging workers in stating that there is some general decline in ability to work with increasing age. They remark, "The physical and mental changes described ... are reflected in a number of studies of job performance ... which have concluded that performance deteriorates with age in a variety of situations that place heavy demands on mental functioning, such as sensory and perceptual activities, selective attention, working memory, and swift information processing. None the less, older workers have a similar productivity rate to young individuals in tasks requiring sustained attention and tasks in which the older workers are highly experienced."

Foggy terminology

There is nothing wrong with such assertions: they are useful guides. But when we have to get practical, do a gerontechnological revamping of a workplace for older workers with a couple of gadgets here, a math model or new interface there, or else we have to design some actual training or reformulate the task, we have some sticky questions to answer: Precisely what is "a heavy demand?" What is "swift?" What is "information," and "processing?" Of course, we all know what such terms mean–but on the other hand, when it comes right down to it, we don't know. These terms can all be operationalized in specific research settings, but then they can't usually be accurately generalized to specific work situations in the field in terms of populations of unspecified older people.

To illustrate further, Giniger, Dispenzieri & Eisenberger (1983) speculated that it could be that older workers are less prone to accidents preventable by judgment than they are to accidents that could be prevented by responding rapidly. This is certainly a worthwhile and useful speculation and seems to make intuitive sense. It gives us a hint of where to look when things go wrong.

But consider the difficulty in nailing these terms down experimentally. Even straightforward concepts such as "Prone to accidents" are customarily very hard to measure in a practical sense, even if this term is rigorously defined in terms of some index such as accident rates on a specific job. Older people report accidents less, so they may appear to be safer than they really are. But, conversely, competent older people who don't tend to have accidents may be promoted so that the accident statistics are derived from their less wily counterparts, so older people would appear to be less safe. Youths who have accidents in some dangerous profession may switch to other professions early on, biasing the sample, and so on. There is the possibility that "accident-prone" may be a characteristic of individual personality. So how can we know?

What is "judgment?" Is it meant to imply somehow that all older people consistently have better judgment in all tasks? Of course not, some do in some tasks some of the time. But can we refine the definition somehow without losing all of its generality? "Responding rapidly" also can't be readily operationalized, defined specifically, especially in the context of some complex accident with serial "domino" components because there are so many attendant variables and immeasurable ones such as the effect of years of mentally preparing for this "freak" emergency.

Perhaps we should also establish a bit of perspective about decline. Most work situations don't really operate very close to the edge of human capacity, so there is room for all kinds of decline. For example, the "biomarker of aging," reaction time, so easy to measure in the laboratory, is one of the measures of performance that is often cited as an instance of something that always declines with age at least in some of its forms. Sometimes it is cited as the only perceptuo-motor component that reliably changes. But, most workplaces, hopefully, don't require low reaction times to insure job performance or safety. (Of course, we exclude some workplaces such as those of the fighting and circus professions: soldiers, jugglers, policemen, firemen, hockey players, lion tamers, and snake charmers.) But even in many of these, technologies allow us to sidestep the demands of vigilance, situational awareness and assessment, decision-making and crisis-driven reaction. And in many cases, such as professional driving, alertness, experience, and forethought can more than make up for factors such as reaction time.

A note of apology to the reader may be in order. On the one hand we are tempted here to include some lists of generalizations like these about older workers for you to think about and write down and remember–"Older workers are more this and less that; they have trouble with tasks involving something or other, and they think about whatever it is 14% less quickly." However, focusing on such findings isn't really accurate or fair, not to older people, nor to you, nor to our own field, nor to the excellent researchers who have derived these general findings. It seems that here of all places we shouldn't contribute to the unrealistic stigmas of age in the workplace.

Moreover, one of the main sources of gerontechnology's power is in the fact that more and more we are able to offer technically specific solutions that offset individual differences in the workplace. As technology burgeons and billows, we are offered the technical flexibility to render the demands of many tasks in the workplace adjustable, adjusting with computers, with training, with robots, with powerful mathematical models and fuzzy sets and neural nets and interfaces.

Some psychological factors to ponder

Satisfaction on the job is related to performance, psychological stress, and attitude toward other employees. Try to think through some sources of psychological impingement. Here are a couple of sources as examples. What would you do about them?

Stigmata from below and above

Stereotyping and stigmatizing has psychological effects. The worker may feel the stigma of increasing age radiating from younger colleagues. There may not be as many things in common. Petty conflicts of territoriality, over the office temperature, the volume of the radio, and preferences in lighting that may well accompany age may be joined by others that are then ascribed to age that may create social rifts. Stigmatism of another ominous sort may also be coming down from a management who knows too well that this one expensive senior's salary will buy them two or three inexpensive new workers, maybe some part-timers: each may be able to out perform and out produce this older "worn out" worker; at least this may be management's dream.

At the extreme, older persons may begin to feel that they don't fit in at work anymore, and these feelings of decreased recognition and esteem at work have been shown to be a significant cause for declining "Work ability index" of Ilmarinen et al. (1997), a general measure related to employability. But, having fit in at work for so long, older people don't fit in anywhere else either. A worker may yearn to leave, but very much be afraid to because there is no acceptable place to go.

Retirement's avalanche of time

Of course, many of us feel that we will know exactly where to go. We await the prospects of retirement with some exuberance because we no longer want to get up too early, drive too far, and work too hard for too many hours burned out on a boring job. We want to get on with that personal project we haven't had time for, we want to volunteer somewhere, and take our trip to Spain. However, the retirement avalanche's torrent of free time is often disillusioning. Retirement may fall far short of being a contribution to health and well-being. Ending 20 or 30 years of dedication to some form of work leaves behind more than just a wastebasket filled with previously important crumbled papers and abandoned pencil stubs in an empty desk. It leaves a personal rubbish heap of once-golden now-useless skills, knacks, facts, company lore, personal connections, benefits, rituals, mannerisms and friendships, a thousand dangling threads of conscious awareness, the coffee machine, the gang: it also leaves an empty pay check, and an empty week filled with structureless days, and then another, and another and another.

A socioeconomic side

Government shares the individual's ambivalent position about retirement. On the one hand, it is sometimes believed in political circles, wrongly, that the country's productivity declines when workers are older. Also, the employment statistics may look better if the young people are occupying the jobs and older people are retired but not counted as "jobless."

On the other edge of it, some governments prefer to spend the retirement funds in other ways, so from that point of view, it is much better to keep older people reporting for work each morning. The tax base profits too if the more expensive older workers are the ones in the jobs paying taxes but this means the industry has to pay these higher salaries, so they have fewer profits to pay taxes on. The political and economic pictures are complex.

As it is in the case of governments, on the industrial side too there is a double-edged sword. Early retirement saves the company or institution from paying the larger salaries of senior workers, but early retirements mean paying bonuses and pensions earlier. One large private company in Finland claims to have saved 5 million Finnish Marks in two years through reductions in the cost of early retirements (Ilmarinen & Louhevaara, 1996). Then, also, there was no longer the loss of experience.

Many companies can't afford the naïveté of younger workers, though on paper the naïveté factor may not appear. It is only the money, the bottom line that jumps out from the administrator's summary on paper.
One company encouraged early retirements and then found that the retirees had banded together on their own and formed other small companies; since

these were so surprisingly successful, the question was heard "Why did we let them leave?" Nevertheless, cutting out those larger salaries is attractive.

"Let them leave" isn't always the scenario. One reason that they leave is legal. Some countries don't have enough jobs for everyone–they may try to clear out room for the new workers by legal means. And there are other reasons. For instance, it is more comfortable for an administration to let an impersonal "policy," wielding age as its justification, force someone out than it is for the administrators to personally convey the decision based on individual personal parameters. Some countries are enacting laws about this type of age discrimination. Meanwhile, there are policies of equal participation in employment for women, minority groups, and others.

How can we apply technology to the senior in the workplace? The five aspects of gerontechnology offer a reasonable but not rigid organizing principle. Once again, these aspects are: Prevention, Compensation, Enhancement, Care, and Research.

Prevention

An ounce of prevention, the queen of gerontechnology's ways in the workplace, is worth a pound of compensation (cure) according to the proverb. So we will discuss it first. Prevention obviates the need for the other four ways that follow it. If we can prevent a problem at work there is no need to enhance the person or enhance the work place, there is no need to compensate for failing functions, no need for care for somebody, and there is less need for research. Thus, prevention reigns as our most important tool over much of the domain of older people at work.
Let's think about prevention in more detail.

What should we prevent?

The list of potential candidates ranges from medical conditions to unproductive effort, to accidents. No doubt you can name twenty things by just thinking about your own workplace, without pausing. To prevent any one of these, we can act in one or both of two spheres–personal or environmental. That is, prevention can be applied to features of older people themselves, or to features of the workplace.

Box 4.2 Japan's "Kaizen" way to help older workers

It is called "kaizen," it is Japan's program for restructuring the workplace for older employees - and it is a keystone of future planning for a nation that already has the longest life expectancy of any place on earth. As with almost every other industrialized society in the world, Japan's population is aging rapidly and, if current rates hold, it will become the oldest on the planet within the next 20 years.

That, reports the American Society on Aging's publication Aging Today, is why the Japanese Government is "paying industry to retool the workplace" to accommodate older men and women, and why it is giving high priority to keeping healthy workers on the job for as long as possible. Thus was born kaizen, and Aging Today gives a couple of examples of how one firm, the Mitsutoyo Company, applied the concept in real-work situations.

It was such successful examples of kaizen, Mitsuo Nagamachi, president of the Kure National Institute of Technology in Hiroshima told a Gerontechnology Conference in Honolulu, which paved the way for Japan's 1998 Employment Security Act for Older People.

As Aging Today explains it, the Tokyo Government under this program offers financial incentives to Japanese firms that hire or retain older workers. "The size of a grant depends on the number of people aged 60 or older working at the company," it added.

According to Aging Today, Nagamachi and his team have come up with a computer-aided system for diagnosing ergonomic problems in the workplace. After an assessment, the Labor Ministry sends a "job-redesign" adviser to the factory, to advise on how to adapt the work sites for older employees.

The researchers say hundreds of factories have already taken advantage of the scheme, and others have expressed interest.

http://www.asaging.org
The American Society of Aging keeps professionals "on the cutting edge in an aging society".

http://www.mediaage.net
MediaAge.net is a news service on aging policies and related issues in Europe.

A staggering array of literature describes the age-related changes in: physical composition of the body, myocardial functions, the respiratory system, cardio-respiratory capacity, musculoskeletal capacity, sensory organs, memory functions, and intelligence. Each of these can interact wildly with assorted factors of the physical and chemical environment at work. So, prevention has bifurcated in response into several avenues of action.

Regulation

We can try to keep people away from harmful influences. The effects of exposure to chemicals in the workplace doubtless change with age. But the exact effects in most cases haven't been assessed. Consider prevention in terms of chemical safety in the workplace, where complex measures have been taken by many agencies and organizations–but not necessarily with much regard for the older worker. Many of the same problems that we encountered in relation to food are here also. It is difficult to test for toxicity because animal models are needed, yet animals usually aren't very good models for humans and even when a good model for a specific toxic agent is found, there is no guarantee that an aged version of the model animal will reflect the sensitivity of an aged person, even though organizations such as the ARBO law (Labor Circumstances Regulations) of the Ministry of Social Affairs in The Netherlands, and the Occupational Safety and Health Authority, OSHA, of the United States have meticulously combed the environments of the workers for hazards and have given great attention to preventing toxic acute or cumulative chemical exposure. Thousands of chemicals that could possibly be inhaled, ingested, drunk, or absorbed or digested into the skin have been categorized in terms of toxicity, maximum allowable levels and times of exposure, symptomology and handling procedures in the workplace.

Theory would suggest that virtually every possible avenue of intake should change with age. For example, absorption through their skins would be suspected to be different in complex ways. First, penetration of chemicals through the skin has been shown to depend on the degree of hydration of the stratum corneum, the 0.1 mm or so of "dead" skin, because water is a strong penetration enhancer: older people tend to have drier skin, but it is thinner. In addition, most recently scientific views of our skin have changed. The skin is not only a passive medium. It is no longer seen as just an inert sheath that only upholsters the body. It performs a wide range of active physiological functions such as xenobiotic metabolism involving metabolizing enzymes specific to the skin (Merk & Jugert, 1993). In a way, the skin is like the stomach: it digests things. Mercury goes in through the skin. The Mad Hatter of Alice in Wonderland was a caricature of hatters of the day whose jobs involved working with mercury. That is a thing of the past, and dentists, who may work with mercury when they fill our teeth, have taken some measures. But, are there other occupations you can think of involving chemicals that should be looked at in terms of toxicity, cumulative or otherwise, to older people?

How about jobs related to the graphic arts with pigments. Let's consider cadmium as an example. Cadmium provides much of the yellow and red color that we enjoy in paintings and pastels. Changes in the heartbeat rate of persons in atmospheres containing as little as 0.002 micrograms per cubic meter of cadmium have been reported. The maximum allowable concentration of cadmium is 100 micrograms per cubic meter!
The issue goes beyond increasing vulnerability or sensitivity. Even if older people aren't more sensitive to cadmium, the effects are likely to be more damaging. For instance, cadmium leads to bone porosity and inhibition of the mechanisms of bone repair–not what they need, and it causes hypertension at very low levels of exposure. Small doses can cause diseases such as pneumonia, which can be more harmful to older people, and colitis. The sources may be subtle. One case was caused from simply drinking liquid stored in a cadmium-plated bowl. It may also be worth noting that older people often turn to painting and other forms of art for amusement.

Rethinking the workplace

Similarly, with respect to the physical working environment, groups such as OSHA, many insurance companies such as Liberty Mutual, and others have examined the physical details of the workplace with minute scrutiny, and have formulated codes for building and maintenance, with the hope of preventing accidents. Falls cost billions of dollars and cause considerable misery in the workplace. Here too, older people require special analysis, which in most cases hasn't yet been accomplished. They have fewer accidents, but the accidents that they do have can be more damaging to them, their modes and methods for avoiding accidents are different, their recovery strategies are too, and the accidents are often of a different sort than younger people have (Laflamme & Menckel, 1995). What is clear is that preventive measures designed for a workplace full of 45-year olds needs to be re-thought, mathematically modeled, and studied from the gerontechnological perspective.

Physical exercise

Other kinds of prevention are simple. We know that cardio-respiratory and musculoskeletal capacity tend to decline with age, but the rate of decline is strongly dependent on the physical activities of the individual (Ilmarinen, 1996). Accordingly, in Japan, many companies conduct sessions of callisthenics for the employees each morning before work hoping to prevent physical problems.

Training

There are two kinds of training that we need to think about, training of specific skills–how to use a personal computer, and life long training.

As an example of the former, there are "back schools" where workers are taught how to lift so that they won't injure their backs on the job. Kovar and La Croix (1987) note that while 58% of the population studied had no difficulty performing the work related activities that were examined, 31% of the women and 15% of the men had difficulty in lifting and carrying a weight of only 10 kg.

Probably, you can think of ten types of short-term training on specific skills that would enhance your own effectiveness as you age on your current or prospective job.

Long-term training has a couple of justifications. Prevention of many problems on the job for older people has to start with training when the person is young. Many of the preventable problems that can be related to aging take years to develop. As noted by Ilmarinen (1996), there is a need to apply preventive measures throughout the entire span of employee ages.

Long-term training, planning in a sense, for eventualities may also be important. If a person's productivity rate begins to fall, it is good if appropriate planning and training over the years has taken place that allows a transition. Then the worker can move smoothly into some other phase of the same job where the years of experience won't be wasted: a fireman can work in dispatch because he/she knows the city, perhaps gradually training for the position while still fighting fires; a ballerina can collaborate in teaching–but you can't just start in and immediately know how to teach, training is required. Any worker should have prior personal involvement in planning what is next and should have the opportunity to train for the transition over an appreciable period of time.

Protection

Presbyacusis, loss of hearing that can begin at a young age with exposure to high levels of sound, is commonly prevented in the workplace by reducing noise levels and supplying and requiring the use of hearing protectors. Older people of an isolated tribe in South Sudan have excellent hearing, even for higher frequency. It is suggestive at least that this is because sounds in their environments seldom exceed 80 dB (Bezooijen, 1996). It is easy to think of other professions where prevention by technological protection could be worked out. How about the professions that subject people to bright flashes of light for example?

Reformulating the job

Prevention by changing the task is sometimes the best solution. The task can be made safer, or it can be made easier along the problem dimensions, or it can be restructured to avoid aggravating the "wear and tear" diseases. Because the average profile of susceptibility to disease of an individual person does change over time, special attention needs to be paid to the changing profiles of older people.

For example, prevalence of osteoarthritis, a disease often having a wear and tear component, increases with age, which suggests certain changes in the work's demands. Avoidance of excessive loading of the joints is important in osteoarthritis, for instance loading by the exertion of heavy force as in playing the piano (Bezooijen, 1996). Similarly osteopenia, decrease in bone strength associated with a decrease in mass, is an age-related disease that

predisposes workers to broken bones. The decrease in cortical bone in older women is 10 to 20% per ten years. What advice would you have for reformulating the job of a jazz piano player? A bus driver? A secretary? Nothing brilliant and highly technical comes to mind? That's fine.
A contribution doesn't have to be either clever or very technical; it just has to make a few annoyances go away.

Early detection, screening

Part of our task here is fairly straightforward: simply adapt the procedures of occupational health care to function well with older workers. Expand the examinations along dimensions that have relevance to their situations. Include more cardiac and pulmonary analyses, check for bone density and the other things that have a tendency to go wrong later in life.

Education

It is one thing to train people on skills so that they won't fall behind and will be able to use the new spreadsheet and the complex graphics program. Education about some of the processes of aging that may impinge on performance is another issue. For example, in driving, tailgating fervently as they always have, many people don't realize that their responses may be slowing a bit. They need to be taught facts like this before they learn the hard way. Actual tests of reaction in a simulator or other convincing demonstrations may help. They may not want to admit that they are slowing–may tail gait even more tightly to prove they aren't, but a few near misses mixed in with the simulator data could prove the point. At least the information is there. If there were standard reaction tests that people were to take every year during their health screenings they could "serve as their own controls" as the psychologists put it: compare present reactions with past reactions to see how things are going. If there is slowing then training about the implications for performing slightly differently on the job could be offered.

> ## Box 4.3 Training for older workers
>
> Collis and Mallier (1998) analyzed the role that government sponsored Training and Enterprise Councils (TECs) are playing in a context where the labor force is aging. Older workers in Britain, and many other countries, are suffering social exclusion as structural and technological changes reduce their job opportunities in an environment of age discrimination. A factor influencing the employability of older workers is the lack of training with which they have been provided. In Britain employers provide little training for workers over the age of 50. For example, only 8% of workers between the ages of 50 and 54 are provided with training by their employers compared with 14% of those aged 20-24. Moreover, recent evidence shows that very few TECs provide training for older workers.
>
> Collis, C. & Mallier, T. (1998). Government and the provision of training for older workers. In: J. Graafmans, V. Taipale & N. Charness. (Eds.). Gerontechnology: A sustainable investment in the future. (pp. 381-384).

Education about the changes that one can expect with age can take many directions. For example, the skin may become drier so things are more easily dropped, and peripheral awareness may diminish so objects in the workspace may be more easily knocked over. What would you recommend for a bartender to offset these two factors?

Prevention is the best solution, but what if the problem wasn't recognized early enough for preventive measures to be applied?

Compensation

The second aspect, compensation, implies that something is already diminished, so performance needs to be refurbished. Perhaps a perceptual skill such as reading is becoming too time-consuming or perhaps a physical task such as shoveling has become too hard. The person simply needs glasses, or a sharper shovel.

There are many common examples of compensation relating the person, per se, which have been devised. These include personal instruments for perceiving such as photogrey eyeglasses, magnifying glasses, hearing aids, and color enhancing schemes. There are many assistive devices such as reachers and grippers, and there are thousands of devices in the form of prosthetics for sensing and knowing. We have also crafted a number of specialized training courses. One of the gerontechnologist's tasks is to stimulate the invention and development of such compensators that enable older workers to continue to perform successfully. And we encourage older people to invent and develop them.

We consider both old and young in compensation too

As it was with prevention, both the younger worker and the older worker have to be considered as candidates, because of the extreme overlap between the groups if for no other reason. In fact, there is evidence that indicates the very young workers may be the ones to perform poorly while older people perform just like everyone else. Mc Evoy & Cascio (1989) have conducted a rather telling survey of the literature on the relation between age of the employee and job performance, which highlights the need for customized compensation. Each person, young or old, has strengths and weaknesses in terms of each kind of job. The old adage still applies, "Don't plow with a racehorse; Don't race with a plow horse."

Mc Evoy and Cascio note, "On the basis of a review of 22 years of articles published in 46 behavioral science journals, we found a total of 96 independent studies that reported age-performance correlations. ... Meta-analysis procedures revealed that age and job performance generally were unrelated. Furthermore, there was little evidence that the type of performance measure (ratings vs. productivity measures) or type of job (professional vs. nonprofessional) moderated the relation between age and performance significantly. However, for very young employees the relation between age and job performance was consistent and modestly positive."

Customization of compensation: age-based or not?

At first thought it might seem that these findings imply it is advisable to adapt the job and its associated equipment for people in the lower tails of the distributions of speed, skill, and the other factors that the job requires. Compensation ideally should accommodate the slowest person, the one with the weakest muscles, the dimmest vision, and the foggiest of memories. But of course this should be done without rendering the job undoable by a person, young or old, with strong muscles, hawk-like vision, and a mind that is crystal clear–and easily bored.

One problem is this: there are many cases where it may be that the slowing senior and the slow beginner are slow for completely different reasons. Then they may require entirely different types of compensation. For example, an aging scientist might profit from some help with memory techniques, whereas a younger scientific counterpart might suffer from lack of knowledge, intuition, and experience.

Also, older people may be capable of utilizing different kinds of compensation by virtue of advanced skill and knowledge gained over the years. The re-designed job could be far beyond the capabilities of a younger worker.

What or who to shore up?

The word, compensation, as we use it here refers to compensation for the older worker's inability to deal with the work situation and does not imply that the person per se necessarily has to be rendered stronger, more intelligent, just more capable of doing the task. Nor does it necessarily mean the job has to get easier. In general, should we be thinking more in terms of the balance between person and task? Often there is an option: either lighten the load or strengthen the person. But, is a tradeoff always possible?

Not always, it depends on the task. Under some circumstances, such as when the task must be highly regimented and structured, compensating for the person's decline may be the only way to keep older people on the same job. Jobs such as copying Morse code, performing simultaneous interpretation of languages, and driving buses are highly event driven. As it is with juggling, thought and action need to be locked critically to the environment. Such tasks are hard to re-design if they can't be slowed, re-structured or simplified very easily. But the envelopes of danger can sometimes be avoided, for example by teaching people not to tail gate. Sometimes parts of the task can be computerized, the control panel simplified or made more ergonomically appropriate. Time and gravity are stern masters. So, in some cases, compensating by training or personal instrumentation may be the only solution.

Other situations may dictate that the compensatory adjustments be applied to the workplace alone. The controls of the weaving machine can be relocated to eliminate long reaching movements, the winch can be power assisted to accommodate the weaker logger, the demands for speed in making executive decisions can be reduced, brighter light bulbs with different spectral distributions can be installed so that counterfeit money is easier for the teller to see, high friction paint can be applied to the ship's deck, and the ship's user interface can be designed to be more friendly.

The situation can be altered

If it isn't feasible to alter either the senior or the job and its context, then the overall situation can still be modified. For example, older people can still be promoted up or transmoted laterally out of the specific job and into a more compatible situation, hopefully one with more status and more money attached to it; one that capitalizes on the person's long years of experience, perspective, and mellowed disposition. Consider one possible modern option for improving the situation of coming to work–don't come to work.

Telework

Presently one of the most extreme possibilities for improving the workplace is a total reformulation of the working environment, teleworking–working from a remote location, such as home. This possibility offers flexibility in scheduling. One can take a nap and work all night, or not work on Friday, and no time is wasted in transit or talking to colleagues about non-essential issues. This may be a particular advantage for older workers or the disabled, who might require intervals of rest or frequent changes in position.

Maintaining and upgrading the levels of compensation

Ongoing "housekeeping by compensation," "tuning" of the workplace is always in order with the specific requirements of the older worker in mind. For instance, older people may be more in danger of having certain specific types of injuries, for example injuries sustained to the back and lower limbs (Laflamme & Menckel, 1995). Improving the workplace in accordance with this finding then might simply mean moving items to be lifted to higher locations so that nothing heavy needs to be lifted from floor level.

It is not difficult to generate long checklists of ways that workplaces and older people that work in them can be altered, and there are countless ways to organize these logically. But for illustration, consider one set of assessments based on the research that has been done.
A WHO study group, based on extensive experiments and observations of researchers in the field (WHO, 1993), presents three groups of ergonomic target opportunities for gerontechnological redesign, training, education, etc., aimed at dealing with premature decline in work capacity among aging workers in relation to "Health Promotion." The WHO groups states:
"The best way of supporting work capacity as workers age is a combination of health promotion and job redesign, taking into account individual needs and ensuring flexibility in the workplace." Accordingly, each of these can be thought of in terms of solutions that enhance either the employee or the environment on a customized basis.

This WHO group emphasizes, "Older workers' needs should always be considered in the design of occupational health and safety programs. In the past these needs have not been given due consideration either at the national level or in practice in the enterprise." The WHO's general recommendations to member states can be summarized as follows: National policies should be adopted by governments and supported by legislation. Policy should encourage "social partners" to enable working well and comfortably into old age. There should be incentives for continuing to work. Employers should be given detailed guidelines for making the workplace compatible with the older worker. Administrators

should be given training in how to accomplish this. Experts, both basic and postgraduate, in the fields of occupational health and safety, nursing, industrial hygiene, ergonomics, psychology, physiotherapy, and safety engineering should be taught about aging and work. More appropriate research is required. Better databases on working older people need to be built. Periodic health examinations should be required after age 45 to test for deficits in strength, performance, and cardio-respiratory functioning which could be improved by exercise. Screening should be carried out for changes in vision, hearing, musculoskeletal facility related to age that would indicate enhancing the person or the workplace.
Healthy lifestyle should be encouraged.

Tailoring the training

Assuming that we can sort out what is trainable from what isn't by experimentation and observation, then it only remains to determine the best ways of training particular skills in order to revamp them. The training sometimes needs to be tailored specifically to older people because it may be necessary for older people to perform certain tasks in different ways. Brute strength may need to be replaced by judgment and cleverness. Also, older people may possess different bases for training than young people do. Especially with respect to computerization of tasks, younger people have knowledge that older people don't–but as always there is a great deal of overlapping variability, some older people may have the knowledge and some youths may. So training may have to be sculpted to fit the individual, trait-by-trait and characteristic-by-characteristic.
Let's consider an example of training on a personal variable–steadiness.

Tremor and training

One of the human attributes that is most basic to working is movement. Difficulties with controlling one's movements such as tremor can invade nearly every aspect of nearly every job. Essential tremor is the most common movement disorder. It has peak prevalence in the sixties and primarily affects the hands and head. Essential tremor can significantly impair performance related to work, communication, household activities, leisure, psychological well-being, and social functioning. Lundervold & Poppen (1995) have developed an overall model for conceptualizing and dealing with tremor in terms of the physiological underpinnings, the physical and social environmental antecedents (trying situations can increase the tremor), level of neural arousal, self-awareness, emotional distress and debilitating self-assessment, all of which influence tremor. Their research suggests that medical intervention, which can bring on side effects that are detrimental to performance at work, can be replaced by simple instruction on relaxation and coping skills and neuromuscular reeducation by biofeedback, at least in the patient group that was investigated.

Training can compensate for many kinds of loss. In areas of mental performance, cognitive training can provide more effective ways of processing information at the workplace to compensate for cognitive slowing. We have mentioned the variability of older people in nearly every context that have been dealt with so far, and here with respect to training we must mention it again. Often methods of training apply to both young and old because of the usual overlap–the fastest, more accurate senior is quite likely to be much faster and more accurate than the slowest or least accurate youth. Further scrambling the two categories, the most alert and well-slept senior may excel over the most groggy and sleepless youth in spite of natural capacities that they each may have. And in fact, depending on the task, older people with their superior experience and intuition and mastery of the job may all outperform the younger workers.

So, as it was in training-to-prevent, and in training-to-enhance, in some kinds of compensatory training young and old can be trained alike. However, there are some well-defined areas where older people need to be trained in very different ways than their younger associates. For example, since older people are usually more frangible because of their lower bone densities and their less elastic tissues they should be trained to fall in different ways than should the young and they should be schooled in ways to stay more to the conservative side of the envelope of probability of falling. Imagine designing some training to compensate for partial loss of vestibular functioning in a roofer? The person has a diminished sense of balance and tends to tip over when the eyes are closed. Would any of the training of airplane pilots to fly in fog apply? How about training of the astronauts with respect to aberrant visual/vestibular signals?

Enhancement

Unfortunately, neither the "use it or lose it" of prevention nor the "train it and regain it" of compensation applied to factors such as muscle strength, will always apply universally throughout aging human performance.
If these fail and the person inevitably loses something valuable from his/her life we look around for ways to give them something else, to provide enrichment, that is, enhancement of what remains of his/her world.

As an example of a possible loss, complex reaction time may slow somewhat as one ages, and may not necessarily be resurrectable by practice or cognitive exercise. In a longitudinal study of visuoconstructive speed, visuomotor speed, and visual search speed, Duvanto et al. (1995) did find such hints of irreversible decline. Nurses and administrators were studied over a long term and it appeared that the demands of high cognitive work on central processes, stemming from their professions, did not prevent a slowing down of the information processing speed with age.

If one were in a profession in which reaction times were crucial, for example piloting commercial aircraft, there might be some point where compensation didn't work well enough anymore and a switch to management or to retirement was necessary. How would enhancement work in this situation? We would assess what is being lost, for instance, social contact. Then we might enhance social contact technologically with the Internet.

Care

When prevention and compensation have not been adequate, an accident has happened and the person involved needs immediate care, or over decades some condition such as an arthritic joint has progressed to the point where it needs attention, the fourth aspect of gerontechnology, care, comes into play.

Older workers may have different conditions

A cut finger is a cut finger for both young and old; however, some of the parameters of care are different for older people in the workplace than for the general worker, depending of course on the specific situations. First, they suffer, probabilistically speaking, from different ailments than the young do. It is true, children with arthritis and diabetes and heart conditions are seen relatively commonly, but these problems are obviously more prevalent in the older population. So at work, emergency care and equipment that encompasses older peoples' profiles of need for emergency care have to be in place. In addition, the workers themselves have to be screened in order to determine what sorts of ailments are represented on the workforce so that the appropriate equipment, procedures, and training can be installed.

Older workers have more conditions that have developed

A second difference between young and older workers is that older workers tend to have more physical conditions that need monitoring and attention. Reporting on the workforce of a large electronics firm in The Netherlands, Durinck (1996) notes, "...it is remarkable that at age 50 many employees are already subjected to unhealthy conditions. Approximately 25% of the workers are already under medical surveillance at the age of 50... This evidence alone brings us to the hypothesis that the age of 50 is too late to start the periodic health examinations. The age of 45 would be more appropriate because it is closer to the actual onset age for disease processes in an aging population."

Box 4.4 Voluntary work

Voluntary work is a forgotten chapter in economics because the work is not translated into salaries or increased national income. From a social point of view, however, it is invaluable and in most countries abundant. If voluntary, unpaid activities would suddenly stop or if all voluntary workers would go on strike, society would be greatly crippled and economics would probably regret its negligence.

Let us describe voluntary work as all organized activities that are being carried out on a voluntary basis and without any payment or with a very low payment in relation to the hours spent. The organizational aspect is crucial, because it refers to the obligation of the worker with respect to others within the organization to carry out the work. The work itself may be secretarial, educational, in the care sector, organizational, or anything else. We exclude here activities for private hobbies or private interest.

One of the difficulties for voluntary work is that the laws and customs governing important protective aspects of professional work such as safety, security, and health do not apply to voluntary work. This leaves the voluntary worker less protected than his/her paid counterpart doing similar work. Next, voluntary work has usually far less training facilities than paid work and for existing training facilities the costs may not be fully covered by the organization. Lifelong learning should be considered a basic achievement of an advanced civilized society rather than an empty slogan.

These difficulties will only be augmented when applied to the senior voluntary workers, whose dispositions may be different, whose health more vulnerable, and whose professional training more necessary, as compared to their younger counterparts.

It seems then that there exists an urgent need to consider these types of problem and find solutions. For as much as the use of technology is involved or can help to solve problems, gerontechnology is in a position to contribute.

Goedhard, W.J.A. (Ed.). (2000). Aging and work 4: healthy and productive aging of older employees. [s.n., S.l.]. ISBN 90-803145-3-6.

The emergencies of older people may require intense and rapid response

A third difference is that older people are more threatened by medical complications so provisions in the care facility for these eventualities need to be established. Monitoring needs to be emphasized more. There is also a need for specialized education in first aid for self help and help by colleagues.

Training

The opportunities for gerontechnology to influence the sphere of care in relation to working fall into three main categories.
First, there is the need for more information about specifics, in even more detail than we have: we have to know what problems that are specific to older people are likely to require care.
Second, better methods of predictive diagnosis have to be derived, which workers require this care?
Third, training programs to encourage and instruct the people who supply the care to shift their attitudes and procedures toward the older worker need to be developed, tested and refined.

Research

The WHO group found that there is a continuing need for more research to assess both the strengths and the needs of the older worker. However, they suggest that the research encompass the full range of working ages and include factors related to modifiable aspects of the workplace and the life style in ways that separate them from the effects of biological aging.

It was suggested that the research should cover theoretical aspects, but also should investigate the validation and evaluation of methods of adapting jobs to suit older workers. This suggests that we will someday have ways to formulate a clear picture of the individual worker to match with a clear picture of the individual job, and we will have well-developed menus of methods for modifying both the individual and the workplace on a highly customizable basis.

Four recommendations of the WHO Study Group

The WHO Study Group recommends to employers, trade unions and regulatory agencies:

1. Work capability, not age, should be the criterion for hiring and retaining employees.
2. There should be flexibility in the design of jobs and the work environment to accommodate the range of the heterogeneous older people and they should have the opportunity to participate in decisions and actions that affect them.
3. Work arrangements should be flexible to allow for job sharing, part-time work and time off for family responsibilities. Part-time work should be encouraged in place of retirement.
4. Every worker should be provided with appropriate education and vocational training as a basic component of work. This education should anticipate technical changes in the workplace and the redesigning of work as workers age, and allow employees to maintain and increase their skills and achieve job satisfaction.

Suggested readings

Charness, N. (Ed.). (1985). Aging and human performance: Studies in human performance. Wiley, New York. ISBN 0-471-90068-0.

Goedhard, W.J.A. (Ed.). (1992). Aging and work 1. ICOH Scientific Committee Aging and Work, [S.l.]. ISBN 90-9005032-9.

Goedhard, W.J.A. (Ed.). (1996). Aging and work 3. ICOH Scientific Committee Aging and Work, [S.l.]. ISBN 90-803145-1-X.

Goedhard, W.J.A. (Ed.). (2000) Aging and work 4: healthy and productive aging of older employees. [s.n., S.l.]. ISBN 90-803145-3-6.

Ilmarinen, J. (Ed.). (1993). Aging and work 2. FIOH, Helsinki. ISBN 951-801-915-0.

Snel, J. & Cremer, R. (Eds.). (1994). Work and aging: a European perspective. Taylor & Francis, Hampshire. ISBN 0-7484-164-4.

WHO Study Group on Aging and Working Capacity. (1993). Aging and working capacity. WHO technical report series no. 835. World Health Organization, Geneva. ISBN 92-4-120835-X.

Suggested websites

http://umetech.niwl.se/SCVN/about_ICOH.html
Website of the International Commission on Occupational Health.

http://www.eto.org.uk/
Website of the European Telework Online.

http://www.occuphealth.fi/e/
Website of the Finnish Institute of Occupational Health.

http://www.osha.gov/
Website of Occupational Safety and Health Administration (OSHA), US Department of Labor.

http://www.uni-ulm.de/LiLL/index.html
Website of the Learning in Later Life network.

CHAPTER FIVE

Personal mobility and transportation

Introduction

Mobility and transportation underlie a broad group of human functions that are important to older people. The rewards of mobility commence each day for the average person with simply getting out of bed, a luxury taken for granted throughout the major part of most lifetimes. Walking in and around the house, and to the bus or car or otherwise traveling, going to the store, to the beach, occupies much of the remainder of the day.

We seldom stop to appreciate the penalties of immobility, nor how life would be even without a small part of our freedoms to move about flexibly. Loss of mobility by a senior can lead to financial decline, inconvenience, depression, and isolation. Gerontechnology tries to stimulate technological activity in each of its five aspects, attempts to discover avenues for dealing with each threat to the conveniences, comforts, and pleasures of walking or wheeling one's self about or using private and public transportation.

Our concerns fall loosely into an assortment of categories, which we note here briefly to stimulate thought, without meaning to suggest rigidly separate domains. There is outdoor mobility, including the use of buses, planes, trains, and cars in contrast with moving about in the house, which has some other sets of problems, a few of which we covered in chapter 3 on housing. Many of these, of course, are in common with problems of moving about outdoors. We can also distinguish mobility that is related to mechanical transportation, cars and buses and such, from walking, and so on.

The anatomy of mobility

Thinking very generally for a moment about the conglomerate of factors that mobility actually is, let us tentatively sketch out some of the specifics that underlie them.

Some of the difficulties are centered on the person. Success at the many components that make up mobility depends on the profile of relevant problem areas that beset older people and we will look briefly at some of the qualities of the individual person, viewed in the specific situation. Skill may be important as may be luck, strength, endurance, alertness, the amount of effort that one is willing to put into the venture, and often the amount of danger or at least fear of it and threat of failure that one is willing to be subjected to. Fear is sometimes justified because if only one link in the chain of events that must take place breaks or is missing, then an entire journey may fail abruptly.

With respect to the person, motor factors would seem to be among the most significant. Could the person walk well and maintain stable posture and balance? How do all the joints and muscles work that are needed movement by movement? Perceptual factors are important too because diminution along the dimensions of vision, hearing, cutaneous sensibilities, and balance have obvious ominous counterparts among the dangers of walking, driving, negotiating a wheel chair, or making one's way to the bus stop (Fozard, 2000). Cognitive facility is of course important because once at the bus stop, you have to know or figure out which bus to get on and know or figure out where to get off. Once in your car, you have to conceptualize and follow a route, and a number of decisions about the actual driving each minute will be based on your mental path on your mental map, so short and long term awareness come into play. In the case of dementia, such as with Alzheimer patients, wandering off and becoming mentally confused is a major consideration that affects many of the decisions related to personal mobility. There are many cases of serious incidents where an Alzheimer patient has driven or walked away. This may be exacerbated suddenly and unexpectedly when the locale is unfamiliar. In Reno, Nevada, a tourist town, an older visitor with Alzheimer's left his family and drove off into an isolated area in the desert, triggering a manhunt lasting many days.
This scenario is relatively common. The strictures and admonishments of childhood may begin to re-emerge and close in on one's mobility.
"Stay close to us, you might get lost."

Mental simulation of aging in mobility–let's pretend

Taking a general inventory of the assortment of behavioral envelopes that constrain the mobility of older people day to day is straightforward. Problems in mobility and the design of solutions can be appreciated and anticipated by applying simple mental simulations. Envision yourself with unbendable knees, as subjects in aging simulation experiments find themselves while wearing leg braces in a simulation of the walking of older people. Or suppose that you have ill-focused vision, or a broken hip. Remain mentally encumbered as you walk in your mind through some set of tasks. Imagine that you have to work at individual jobs that challenge the specific handicap, you are a postal worker, then a watchmaker. Imagine that you have to leave a burning building, or chase a criminal. Could you perform your present job with hazy vision? Try it in your mind and a host of difficulties that may not have occurred to you may present themselves. Could you go to dinner at your friend's house if you had only half of your present physical power to grasp and hold on to the doorknobs, silverware, crystal glassware, the gravy bowl, and other objects; could you go to the opera where the stairs are so steep and dark? Another way to visit some of the frustration of older people who has become less mobile is to just imagine being randomly confronted with the normal things in life that you can't do very well.

Prevalence of lowered mobility

How widespread are these problems? Their seriousness must be weighted in accordance with current statistics about mobility and transportation of older people. Of course, "lack of mobility" is a classification with arbitrary boundaries that depend wholly on the choice of definition. Nevertheless, some general idea of the extent of the problem can be gleaned from assertions of agencies that deal in this area. For example, mobility impairment affects 60 to 80 million people in the European Union according to the TIDE office (Technology Initiative for Disabled and Elderly People). The percent of the population that are in any sense disabled is estimated to be between 17 and 22%. Two-thirds of the disabled are over 60, and 30-50% of the people over 60 have a disability.
Depending on which country we focus on, a significant number of people may draw disability pensions related to losses in mobility.
In the Netherlands, between 1990 and 1994, 282,000 people 55 and older had to use some form of aid (such as canes, other persons and wheelchairs) to get around. Four hundred and twenty-five thousand of those over 55

couldn't walk 400 meters without taking a break. So, on the average, although most older people are quite mobile, the problem demands attention.

Another issue is important. More and more seniors are driving. In addition to its other implications, this means that more and more older people will have to stop driving eventually, after having hinged many important details of their lives on the automobile. In the United States in 1994 there were about 16 million older drivers, a 45% increase over the number ten years previous to that, whereas the total number of drivers increased by only 13% during that same period (U.S. Department of Transportation, 1994).

Statistics such as these shed light on the less mobile members of the general population. But, they tend to miss the mark in some ways by focusing on one category of chronically demobilized people. This obscures the fact that nearly everyone, eventually, for some period of time, will become immobilized to one degree or another and will need to draw on the advances that will have been accomplished in these areas.

So thinking and action about the problems shouldn't be restricted to the plight of a small group of older people sitting in wheelchairs because there are also the people with sprains and broken bones, recuperation from the operating room and other periods of temporary loss of mobility that belong more fleetingly to the same category. These shorter periods not only immobilize the victim, they may cause deconditioning which can threaten other factors relating to health and thus cause more permanent losses of mobility in a circular fashion. Spirduso (1995) characterizes this spiral as, "The vicious cycle of declining mobility caused by sedentary living."

Some current questions

Simulating dangerous situations and modeling the domains of movement mathematically is very important. Why? On one side because falling is so significant to older people because of the damage, yet the dynamics of falling are so terribly hard to characterize and control. For instance, most falls at work, and presumably many of the falls that occur elsewhere, occur on level footing that appears normal. There are similar puzzles in driving. In two-vehicle fatal crashes involving an older driver and a younger driver, the vehicle driven by older people in one study was 3.6 times as likely to be the one that was struck. Why? A few of the reasons are easy to identify: turning into danger unseen because of glare, stopping inappropriately, the youths were driving too fast, and so on. But in the actual fabric of variables related to traffic, what, in minute detail, does such a finding imply that we should change, if not about the older driver, then about the context that the older driver has to drive in? We have to model to unveil the answers. To enhance the data base for the models, we should initiate minutely detailed senior-oriented assessments of the participants in accidents and the associated data on difficulties ranging from small inconveniences, to near misses, to accidents.

The ethical side–mobility: Who gets it? Who pays?

When are you too old to drive? Never? At forty? When are you too young to drive? It's a question with many of the same puzzles. When should we decide that someone's situation is so demanding that public transportation can no longer be made available?

The answers to questions such as these are arbitrary, pick a number. But once we make a choice, we are faced with the responsibility of backing our choice up with technology, thought, and money. There is no clear-cut reason that we shouldn't start driving at ten, but then we need to revamp the training and maybe change the highways some.

Neither is there any logical reason to remain preoccupied with the issue of age in driving. However, there are some practical reasons related to two things: cost and public safety. In driving, capability depends on the type of driving, on one's own attitudes, aptitudes, abilities, and so on. If the truth were known, none of us should be driving; we are all hazards to the public and menaces to ourselves. But each of these factors, attitude and so on, can be shored up by training, screening, ad campaigns and the rest of it.
Each new level of sophistication costs money: when does the effort stop being worth it? Any thoughts on how to make these decisions? How do you feel that this cost/benefit balance should be handled with respect to indoor mobility?

Activity in the five aspects

As before, first we encourage prevention of the problems of mobility for the aging. If we can't prevent, we compensate and return mobility back to its previous levels, or better, by tuning up either the person or the environment. When enhancement of specific skills and equipment for mobility is too difficult then we look for technology that can enhance the home environment to reduce the need for mobility. If that too fails and personally-managed mobility won't work, then we find technology to "care," take charge of the person's mobility using free rides and other tools, so that even at this point, though there may still be loss of mobility as it was once experienced, at least there will be no losses in the advantages that mobility provides.

The technique of prevention

The method of prevention in mobility has followed each of us practically from our beginnings as humans, with increasingly complex rules over our passing years. It started out simple, and got impossible, "Don't drag your feet or you'll trip, don't leave your toys on the stairway or Grandma will trip, stop look and listen, leave one car's length of space between your car and the car ahead for every ten miles per hour of speed, yield to the right unless... ." Disaster-driven folk-research has churned out many of the guidelines that we use for safe mobility, and these usually have been serviceable, if superstitiously grounded.

Prevention begins with assessment

Before we can prevent, we have to know what needs to be prevented–what irritations, impediments, and dangers are imminent? What are the characteristics of older people and their worlds that make them fall when they walk, beside the obvious things such as dragging the feet?
What hazards make them trip so often when they don't drag them?
Why don't some of them see oncoming cars sometimes? When does it happen? What regions of the environment are the most dangerous in terms of accidents of locomotion? How can we best alert the senses to warn of the dangers in locomotion?

Generating this data for assessment is easy, or at least it is straightforward. A great deal of careful thinking and analysis has already been combined with data and experience from the past about older people and data from the psychophysical and engineering research laboratories. A database is being developed and models, verbal, physical, and mathematical, for why older people have accidents of mobility are being worked out. Many groups have become involved.

One good example of assessment in prevention falls into the category of screening. Recently Ball and Owsley (1995) have developed a system for measuring the "useful field of view" (UFOV), which encompasses both visual attention and cognitive processing speed. They found that drivers with reduced UFOV were 16 times more likely to have been involved in a crash during the previous five years than those without reductions. It is at least suggestive that UFOV can decline with age. Augmenting safety by a factor of 16 is very much worth pursuing and developments of this kind can be quite important to safe mobility. Where can technology come in? Can we change their fields of view or make UFOV less important in the task of driving?

There are many more frontiers of assessment. The literature, and the Internet, can be turned to for the details of research. Please, don't conclude from the immensity of the mountain of research that there is nothing left for you to do. It may seem that every conceivable research question is being addressed, but in fact it is only a small beginning.

It is impossible not to be awed by this maelstrom of activity. Literally thousands of grants are being funded around the world, there are dozens of conferences being conducted yearly that focus at least in part on the senior in transit, and many additional surveys are being carried out to gather more information.

Gerontechnology has a difficult job in looking for ways to assure that all of this information becomes integrated into monolithic packages, theoretical, mathematical, or utilitarian, that encompass the mobility of older people in meaningful ways. Then, how can we funnel the information to where it is needed?

Prevention as education of seniors

Once information is reformulated to suit the problems and the people and the situations, it must be implemented. Implementation may take the form of simply training older people to use the findings in whatever form they may be, cautions, rules of thumb, suggestions. Then the task is to put the information into the minds and memories in forms that will be interpreted correctly and will lead to good reflexive responses in complexly dangerous situations. If this is the aim, then findings have to be condensed, then simplified, mnemonized–cast into a form in which they can be remembered, and finally publicized or taught.

Alternately, we can build machines or environments and teach them the information instead

The intelligence that science derives can often be placed into assistive machines instead of people. Modern technology in the form of computerized interfaces to global positioning systems and other aids to guidance, locators, or even the primitive technology of compasses, has amazing potential. Devices can be incorporated into modules that can be enormously helpful to seniors, can be deployed in and around their cars and in shoes and canes and on the "dash boards" of their walkers.
This of course brings us back to education, imparting instructions and providing practice in using the devices.

When do older people need special preventive training?

Again using mobility in traffic to illustrate, if there were only a few seniors driving, at first thought it would perhaps be easiest to simply incorporate them into the general group of drivers needing further training. They may be slowing and perhaps losing some peripheral vision, but there is still a great deal of overlap with the younger drivers. Also, there are ample studies showing that age, per se, doesn't necessarily predict bad driving (except in the case of the very young). It's more a matter of conditions that may become more serious with age, not the age itself. So perhaps in some ways at least it is feasible to group them together for training and not think about age at all. This is often done in the case of disability.

Box 5.1 Citizen's network

The European Commission has suggested the development of an integrated "Citizen's Network" to make public transport more attractive and usable.

A number of features have been specified. The thinking is based on overall considerations of what it takes to get a traveler from door to door. This goal is achieved in some sense most fully by the private automobile; however parking makes the taxi a more attractive alternative; but individual taxis are too expensive, and so on. So the aim is to provide parts of people's journeys, integrated to make them seamless. For example, even though a trip might involve a taxi, a bus, and then a train, only one ticket need be purchased. Some operators arrange for taxis to interchange passengers with buses. In some places "night buses" will stop directly in front of a person's house. In other countries it is possible to buy a train ticket that includes a "train taxi," at a reduced rate. Such a taxi may be shared by a number of people, so a bit of time may be sacrificed, but at least the journey can be door to door. Multi mode facilities are being constructed elsewhere. Then a train or bus station may become not only a train and bus station, but also an enclosed parking facility for automobiles, storage and rental facility for bicycles and scooters, and a subway station and perhaps an airport.

Baggage presently is a factor that keeps many older people home, so the ideal integrated system will have to encompass that somehow. The suitcases are heavy, especially important if stairs or entry into trains is involved. Bags can be stolen, or forgotten. In addition to transporting older people seamlessly, we need to develop a good system of door-to-door check in. Your ticket not only includes all of the taxi, train, plane and bus fares. Someone shows up at your door to take your suitcase to the plane, train, or bus and check it in, and perhaps take you, without requiring extra money–and tipping is strictly not allowed. You won't see your baggage again until a delivery person carries it into your house. No older person should ever need to lift a heavy suitcase from the baggage carousel and onto a cart (which may not even be available), haul it up the stairs or juggle it onto the escalator and then lift it into the trunk of a car or hoist it into a bus.

European Commission. (1996). European Commission Green Paper.
The citizens' network: Fulfilling the potential of public passenger transport in Europe. COM(95), 601final.
http://europa.eu.int/en/record/green/gp9601/ind_cit.htm

On the other hand, some findings tentatively can be interpreted to mean that there should be special considerations with respect to the older drivers. For example, as previously noted, according to the U.S. Department of Transportation Traffic Safety Facts 1994, cited above, "In two-vehicle fatal crashes involving an older driver and a younger driver, the vehicle driven by older people was 3.6 times as likely to be the one that was struck. ... In 28 percent of the crashes the older driver was turning left–9 times as often as the younger driver." The task in a left turn involves a sudden increase in complexity from simply staying within the lane to attending to additional vehicles, estimating their speeds and distances that will be traveled and estimating one's own velocity and time required to cross in front of the other vehicles.

One factor that sets older people apart is "perceptuomotor surprise." Seniors learned to walk, and drive, with pristine young neural and ophthalmic equipment and formed many automatic habits of performance and judgment. Their characteristics may decline so slowly that the decline isn't even noticed. But the deficits may exert their critical contributions abruptly. As with the surprise of threading a needle, with trembling hands and fuzzy vision at an advanced age if one hadn't sewn since childhood, a motorist whose reaction time has increased slowly over the years might never know that it has changed, nor know that the safe distance for following the car ahead had doubled for him/her, until the driver ahead one day suddenly slams on the brakes. Older drivers have the store of knowledge, wisdom, and experience that younger drivers lack; they only need to be alerted to their need for different strategies in driving and walking. Clearly, older people do need to be trained differently sometimes. However, most of their needs for preventive measures match those of everyone else. We all need to be able to see the lines on the highway better in the rain, follow other cars less closely, and have many other needs for education in common.

The second facet: Compensation

As with prevention, often the political focus obscures the distinctions between compensation for young and for old. The goal in some spheres is simply one of compensating for the general abilities of "people" who have difficulties in mobility. This is good in some ways.
Then older people are not singled out, further stigmatized, and it isn't necessary to deal with two groups: disabled and disabled older people.

However, as we have realized before, there sometimes may have to be a bit of senior customization. It is easy to think of many situations where improving the circumstances for the young might not help the old, might even make things worse for them, and visa versa. The old need to fall differently; they have different mental and physical assets for recovering from threatening situations in traffic, and so forth.

The ADA–Compensation in the environments of old and young

Consider one representative approach, that of the United States. "Disability" has been swept into one basket and everyone is championed and legally guaranteed their rights to be mobile by a single legal mechanism, the Americans with Disabilities Act (ADA).

"An individual with a disability is defined by the ADA as a person who has a physical or mental impairment that substantially limits one or more major life activities..." In this sweeping definition, mobility of older people is mixed in with the mobility of the young.

"Mobility" under this legislation is regarded as being modular, as having separate components, such as guaranteed safe access to facilities and other architectural standards when the modifications that are necessary can be made without "undue hardship." Discriminating with respect to age or not, these efforts have been impressive and heartening.

Many governments have offered assistance

In other countries as well there has been activity designed to improve the transportation environment. A Eurolink Age seminar in Brussels, in 1993 brought together a number of discussants who highlighted the following advances in enhancing the environments of older people throughout Europe: The European Union has taken a number of actions in favor of "older and disabled" persons (Eurolink Age, 1994). In Dublin, the Action for Mobility program operates on the principle of not isolating older people or people with disabilities from others.
"Older people should not be treated in isolation as a special case…"
Sweden has the intermediate transport system, which has spread elsewhere, e.g. the London weekly shopping service.

Similarly laudable, there is the Grenoble tramway and the fully accessible Underground in Lille. Munich Metro is "accessible" as are many others. Standards have been drawn up for accessible buses, there are talking bus stops in Brittany that allow the impaired passenger to communicate directly with the driver and there are many other special bus services. For example there is the free Berlin Telebus service available to disabled and to people over 80 without disabilities, serving 18,000 people and supporting 660,000 journeys each year. Eighty buses are equipped with radios and ramps or lifts and drivers receive special education. The Swedish Service Bus offers a flexible timetable over a flexible route and only costs 10% more to operate than the normal service. Increasingly, taxis are being seen as the most cost-effective way of providing a 24-hour door-to-door service. Subsidized taxi schemes operate in Germany. Similarly, there is the Taxi-card service in London, which allows one roundtrip journey per week. The Eurotaxi service in Spain also uses vouchers supported by the county and the province.

Railways have been revamped too. In 1992 there were 1,000 to 1,300 people in wheelchairs using the Gare du Nord rail station in Paris each month. All the TGV high-speed trains are accessible to wheelchairs in France. The Netherlands provides tactile guide ways in the pavement that you can feel through your shoes, and two-way speaker systems at ticket offices.

Box 5.2 Technology and the bicycle

Bicycling is a healthy mode of transportation that in principle is excellent for older people. There are several advantages to bicycling. You can do it at your own speed. It provides door-to-door mobility with no parking problem and no depreciation nor maintenance. You can carry things that would be too taxing to carry by hand because the bicycle instead of you fights gravity, and yet you get physical exercise. Disadvantages of course are several. You are exposed to the influences of weather. You can take along at the very most two friends. It can be dangerous to use your bike in busy traffic, your balance becomes an issue, and the physical demands can be too great, especially if the terrain isn't relatively flat. Still, people are able to use their bicycles until very old age. In the Netherlands, where bicycling is very popular, 30% of the men above 65 and 55% of the women own bicycles. Here, the mean distance traversed by bicycle decreases significantly only after 75 yrs. (CBS 1997).

Age group	30-40	40-50	50-60	60-65	65-75	75+
Men	2.88	2.77	2.66	2.85	2.66	1.75
Women	2.82	2.76	2.44	2.53	1.89	0.82

Figure 1. Mean distance (in km) traveled by bicycle per day in 1996 in the Netherlands.

A revolutionary new product, called TransGlide 2000™ (by BTS Inc., Denver) can stimulate the use of bicycles by older people by providing a supportive, more comfortable environment. This is a system where bicyclists in a corridor, on safe separate lanes, are supported by air that is moved through the system in the same direction as the bicyclists are riding. This removes the greatest resistance that a bicyclist must overcome and makes bicycling 90% more efficient.
This system is a powerful example of the use of well-established technology for an idea that could meet a demand of older people.

A device such as a bicycle has the potential to virtually bristle with assistive technology to keep the user riding. For example, how about bicycles that let down side supports, outriggers, when you slow to below a certain speed, for instance on stopping for a traffic light. This would obviate the need for putting down a foot when stopping, one precursor of tipping over.

http://www.biketrans.com/index.html

The same general considerations have been extended to access to commercial airplanes and to the facilities inside the plane. However, one weak link in a transport chain is enough to make a whole journey impossible, even render all long journeys impossible for some people. For instance, flight attendants give wheelchair rides to people who need them and all manner of special considerations–alas, so near to transportation, but yet so far: the wheelchairs won't ordinarily fit in the aisles of the plane itself, though some airlines do have narrow versions just for getting the person off the plane and onto a normal wheel chair. Still, of course, no wheel chair could fit inside the locker-sized toilets.

Solutions to such problems often require a different way of thinking, even to the extent of dictating different infrastructures. The "fast as possible" demands from technology that challenge older people, trains that stop for one minute, "Hurry up" signs, busses that don't kneel and brisk timings such as we find in "Walk" signals should all be targets.
Compensation in mobility also extends to the terrain, the sidewalks and the streets; and it should. In the United Kingdom 45 percent of all fatalities involve older pedestrians. Town planning should take into account the risk of dangerous pavements. In the Netherlands 7,000 pavement accident victims a year need medical treatment.

Changing aspects of the person rather than the environment

Training, augmenting the mind, is often easier than changing the surroundings or the physiology of the person. There are a number of excellent beginnings in this direction.

Training of mental style and attitude in driving or walking

In a study on the effects on braking response time of collision warnings given to older and younger drivers, Vercruyssen and his associates (1996) found that when braking in response to an auditory or visual warning, or in response to "deceleration" of a car "in front" (in a simulator), it was not only the complexity of the task that affected the older driver, but also the driver's state of arousal.

Box 5.3 Smart roads

For older people the automobile is a principle means of transportation. Intelligent Transportation Systems (ITS) or telematics have much to offer. ITS is a broad area that includes near-term and long-term ambitious applications of advanced technologies. Automated Highway Systems (AHS) is an area under ITS that promises to dramatically improve the efficiency and safety of the current highway system. In AHS technologies will be integrated to produce a highway system where fully automated vehicles are guided to their destinations and the flow of traffic is controlled and optimized for maximum efficiency and safety. It will take 20 to 30 years before a complete automated system is realized. Highways will be similar to air traffic routes, with a central Traffic Control that channels the cars to avoid traffic-jams and collisions. Automation of the driving task will compensate for the decreasing capacities of older people, increase safety and stimulate mobility.

Several concepts and products already operate successfully:

Advanced Traveler Information Systems (ATIS). The RDS/TMC system (Radio Data Systems/ Traffic Message Channel) provides broadcast information about road and traffic conditions. ATIS also includes on-board route guidance systems to help motorists find their way.

Advanced Vehicle Control Systems (AVCS). AVCS includes a broad range of products that enhance the driver's control of the vehicle. These products include collision warning systems, detection of objects in the blind spots, collision avoidance using automated braking and/or automated steering, intelligent speed adaptation, intelligent cruise control, and so forth.

Older users of AHS hopefully will feel that it is a better, more comfortable and safer way of driving, if not too many new tasks are added to the driving task and if the characteristics of older people are taken into account in the development and design process. Potentially AHS can increase the sense of security and independence, and support a life-style that increasingly depends on mobility.

Ioannou, P.A. (1997). Automated highway systems. Plenum Press, New York. ISBN 0-306-45469-6.

Slowing with age was observed across tasks; however, when drivers were prepared and alert, age differences were reduced considerably. This implies that at least some factors that are within the driver's control, such as alertness, can elevate the level of safety and suggests that drivers may simply need to be reminded from time to time of the importance of attitude and vigilance. The car could even monitor and test its driver and remind him/her as required to be vigilant. Can you think of some ways of doing this? In-vehicle technology of this sort is being developed in the field of Intelligent Transportation Systems.

In driving and walking it is often important to share one's mental time between the various tasks, the footing, a sign board, another pedestrian, back to the footing, and so on. In studying the effects of age and expertise on the efficiency of time-sharing, Tsang and Shaner (1998) found that time-sharing efficiency declined with age, but "expertise in time sharing appeared to be able to moderate some of the deleterious effects of age." What sort of training program might we use to capitalize on this trainability of attentional skill?

Compensation provided by self-monitoring

One promising direction for improvement of performance is in educating the person about him/her self. The American Automobile Association Foundation for Traffic Safety has redesigned its popular self-assessment tool for older drivers, "Drivers 55 Plus: Check Your Own Performance." This self-test helps mature drivers improve skills.
Well over 130,000 copies of this document have been distributed since 1986. The fifteen-question test developed by Malfetti and Winter, together with Schieber, requires drivers to rate comfort level when dealing with common traffic situations.

The American Association of Motor Vehicle Administrators offers a catalogue of printed and audio-visual materials that deal with older drivers. The listing includes a number of popular pamphlets drawn from the American Automobile Association, the American Association of Retired Persons, and the insurance industry. In North America, some state and provincial handbooks for drivers include specific reference to older drivers.

Texas makes available pamphlets that tell older drivers how to recognize and adjust to age-related changes in physical and mental condition. There are pamphlets advising the older person on options, such as graduated licensing and they even encourage doctors to issue "prescriptions" for people to enroll in older-driver safety courses. All of these help a person to see their skills for driving more objectively.

The American Association of Retired Persons (AARP) produces a booklet for older drivers that includes questions related to the probability that the person will have an accident (AARP, 1992). This represents an excellent application of technology, in non-technical terms, to the driving performance of older people. It is worth some time here because it represents one of the directions that gerontechnology encourages in applying technical information and concepts to older people.

Some of the questions that are asked in the booklet are: How often do you drive? Do you drive at night? Have you experienced frequent or unusual memory problems over the last year? In the last three years, have you had any traffic accidents or traffic violations?
Each of these is correlated with risk of an accident.

Also included are self-tests that determine where the individual falls in terms of national norms. For example, the test on reaction time (actual perception, cognition, and performance time) is a photograph of a traffic scene. Fourteen small numbers are placed in random-appearing locations within the scene. The reader is to touch these numbers in ascending order as quickly as possible, trying to touch as many as possible in ten seconds. (An alternate approach that is easier to perform alone is to simply touch them all and then look at one's watch to determine how much time was taken. The number that would have been touched in ten seconds is then easy to calculate.)

The older person is able to compare his/her performance with that of people of different age groups. The average number of target numbers that can be touched by people 17 years old and under in the ten seconds is 12 to 13. The average for people 70 and over is 6 to 9. Below, for illustration only since there is no standardized data available, a similar test is constructed to convey the general feel of the situation to you. How long does it take you to touch the 14 numbers in order?

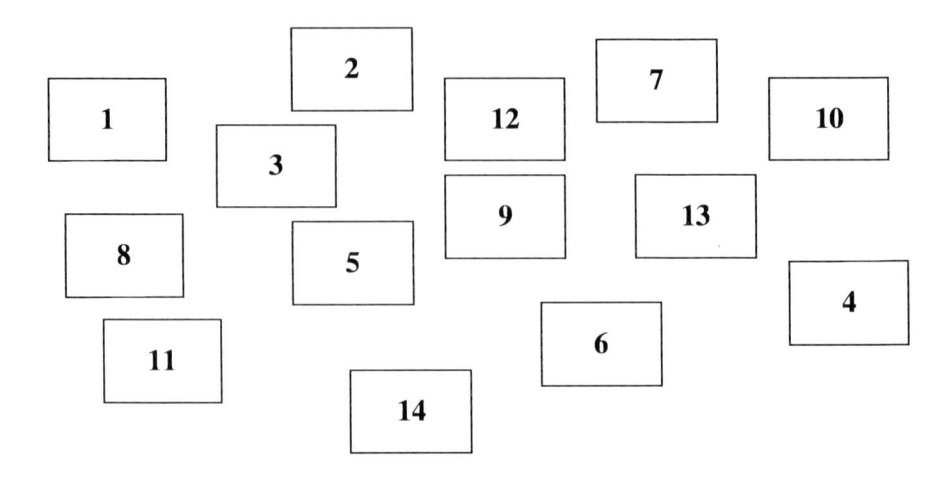

Figure 5.1 Self-test on speed of reaction

The AARP's questions also implicitly instruct about the dangers of distraction by asking questions about attention: Do you talk with your passengers while you drive? Do you smoke while you drive? Do you drink coffee while you drive? Do you eat while you drive? Do you listen to the radio while you drive? Do you watch the scenery while you drive? Do you use your car phone while you drive? There are also rough but effective simulations of some of the perceptual effects that may accompany aging. The phenomenon of shrinkage of one's attention window is illustrated through pictures and its size in relation to factors such as personal stress is shown pictorially.
Questions about vision are asked, and two vision charts, one of high contrast and the other of low contrast, washed out, are provided so that the older person can test him/her self and can appreciate the effects first hand.

History of accidents has been shown to be a warning sign; therefore questions are asked about close calls, actual accidents and abrasive experiences in traffic. Do others honk at you? After driving, do you feel physically exhausted? Do intersections bother you because there is so much to watch for in all directions, and so on.

Attitude of the driver has been shown to relate to performance in driving, so the reader is asked about agreement or disagreement with two types of statements, for example, "Driving with no accidents is mainly a matter of luck," in contrast with, "The very careful driver can prevent any accident." It is pointed out to the older person that people who agree with statements of the first type do tend to have more accidents. Throughout, tips on improving driving skill are given. Finally, there is an assessment and suggestions for improving the chances of remaining accident free; for example, the suggestion that the older person might want to take a refresher course by enrolling in the AARP's "55 Alive/Mature driving" program, an eight-hour classroom course.

Technology for compensation in driving

Today we are just trying to approach the problem of compensation in traffic with larger signs, rumble strips, speed bumps, better lane markings and advance warnings of stoplights. However, our technological development is moving toward more sophisticated solutions, for instance, smart cars and smart highways. Smart cars will be able to compensate for restricted fields of view, restricted neck mobility and restricted peripheral awareness by monitoring positions and movements of cars to the fore, behind and to the sides. They will either monitor themselves, or the highway will do it–know where each car is and what it is doing.
Smart cars and smart highways potentially can carry on continual discourse about either the highway's or the car's time-varying database of traffic velocities, directions, densities and hazards.

The third approach: Enhancement

If some part of one's freedom of mobility is actually lost and compensation can't bring it back, how can the individual still find satisfaction? What commodities will be satisfying in place of mobility?

Pieces of mobility

In the court systems there is the realization that much of what a person loses in fact can't be replaced. The court doesn't know what will satisfy the victim, everyone is different, so it does the best thing that it can do. Though it may seem crass, especially in some cases, the recompense for a damage that is given is simply money–let the individual victim decide what will fill in the missing pieces best. Of course, money, per se, actually has nothing to do with it. The money only represents flexibility–it represents a host of options in the form of what the money will buy. So what is the currency of mobility? What are its individual parts? What are the personal reasons that people want mobility? In short, what do we need to compensate them for?

All motion is relative

The first thing that may come to mind, tautological as it may sound, is that they move about to arrive at things that are in some other location. To this we might counter with the quote, "If Mohamed won't come to the mountain, bring the mountain to Mohamed." What mountains do we need to worry about bringing? First are the necessities of survival. Groceries, heat, and water. The chances are that we are already bringing water, and fuel oil or natural gas for heat to the person. Many locales have set up Meals on Wheels, and ways of ordering and delivering groceries.
The Internet will make this even more satisfactory because the continually updated inventories of stores will be available to the immobilized senior, on-line, as the menus of many restaurants presently are.

Because it's there

One commodity, however, is more difficult to deliver: that mysterious and ill-defined reason for going out known only as, "Just to get out." Presumably this can be dissected too, perhaps into stretching one's muscles, having fresh visual scenes to look at, and having something to look forward to. Of course, there are the exercise bicycle and the television, respectively, to satisfy the first two desires.

Wheatstone about one hundred fifty years ago proclaimed, after he had invented the stereoscope for viewing pictures of scenery in realistic three dimensions that now there would no longer be a need for people to travel. It would seem that we could expect the amazing interactive realism of virtual reality to take us nearer that ideal. Video games for the younger set compensate for some of the needs for self-testing and adventure.
What would video games for older people need to supply? We need a psychophysics of entertainment, and of restlessness for older people. Any ideas?

Mobility for communication

Another of mobility's contributions to living is in allowing people to go here and there to talk to other people, to go over and help peel the potatoes and play with the grandchildren. Why? Because of the good feelings that it gives, and because of the bad feelings that it keeps away. People need good feelings: they may become frightened without them. Do we then need to research the psychophysics of joy, of self-importance and the other sacred human emotions so these can be compensated for–substituted? Or would that be beyond the boundaries of discretion and privacy?

The fourth aspect: Care

When some segment of mobility fails and the older person is confined to the house, or at least, when mobility is momentarily suspended for some reason, gerontechnology invests its efforts in the fourth aspect. Then active and passive alarms, fell-down alerts automatically calling out over the phone to the hospital, and all of the trappings of domotics and telematics come to bear.

I just need a place to sit down

The term, care, in the context of transportation, doesn't need to conjure up visions of ambulances and hospitals. Care in terms of simple needs qualifies. We can invent a better hospital bed maybe, or a better way to get from the bed to the wheelchair while that leg is mending. One interesting device for personal mobility that has been evolving out of the care arenas of the medical wards and into the supermarkets is a version of the old standby, the "walker," with its physically and psychologically cold polished aluminum frame for grasping and its small wheels that could only be meant for the smooth floor in the hospital.

Now we are beginning to see gaily-colored frames sportily appointed with nice big wheels, big enough even for cobblestones! On looking closer one sees a hook in the front for hanging shopping bags; there is also a basket for carrying groceries around in the store or for stowing personal items that might be needed on an outing around the lake. But where does the care come in? There is a foldout seat that you can sit on when you are tired!

The fifth line of effort: Research

Study situations more than individual variables

There is a general principle that is important when studying the mobility of older people. Research in psychophysics and engineering laboratories is very valuable for some purposes, but there are problems. Because of the rigid control of variables and the smoothing of the data to get at underlying phenomena through the noise, data doesn't always transplant well to the outside world when it comes to mobility of older people. We often find that the data isn't representative of the real world.

Dangerous situations usually involve interactions in concert of the person and the environment where the relevant variables are numerous and complexly tangled together. In planning for safe design, or investigating an accident that has already happened, it is important to somehow acknowledge and accommodate all of the possible dangerous combinations of the factors.
Further, it is necessary to think along hypothetical time lines–envision all possible chains of action/reaction sequences. Virtually all accidents related to mobility are "freak" and bizarre: many can happen only when several dangerous factors combine simultaneously. Pure coincidence of events can be the factor that causes trouble so all possible coincidences have to be foreseen. Glare from the sun may not be a problem, until it obscures the trip hazard at exactly the time of day when a person is walking over it, or suddenly dazzles the eyes through the rearview mirror.

Unpredictable chaining of actions and subsequent reactions can cause unpredictable accidents. It may not be the initial slip of the foot, but rather the subsequent slip by the opposite foot on a surface where this second foot, recovering from the first slip, was never anticipated as being by the designer of the building, nor the contractor, nor the foot's owner.

Chains of mental events support much of personal mobility. It may be that a long series of distractions while the victim was walking all combined with some slippery spilled liquid. Perhaps the inadvertent turning of the steering wheel while digging in the glove box for some gumdrops led to a mild over-correction, which called for more and more analysis of the traffic until some targets of attention simply had to be passed over.

An older person might well recover from one segment of a sequence, but the effects of serial threats can be multiplicative, successively straining the resources until they fail.

One of the technological tools that applies immediately to complex situations is again mathematics. For instance friction, and visibility, and reaction time, and force, and acceleration and the rest have all been measured for virtually every place that a person might walk or drive. But in complex situations of the type that real accidents are made from, simple two- and three-dimensional relationships are likely to be invalid and not representative of the actual situations.

Mathematical models of locomotion as it occurs in all the various realms of mobility are needed, together with the psychophysical experimentation that is required. It is necessary to discover the forms of the models and define their parameters and fill them out. All of this needs to be embodied in computer programs that can assess situations that surround mobility and warn us of problems that may catch up with people in the future. Devices need to be programmed and attached to us here and there–older people can benefit from smart shoes, smart canes, smart walkers, smart crutches, smart cars, smart stairs, and smart bicycles.

Suggested readings

Elias, J.W. (Ed.). (1994). Experimental aging research, 20, 1, Special issue devoted to aging and driving. Taylor and Francis, Washington D.C. ISSN 0361-073X.

Fozard, J.L. (2000). Sensory and cognitive changes with age. In: K.W. Schaie & M. Pietrucha. (Eds.). (2000). Mobility and transportation in the elderly. (pp. 1-44). Springer Publishing, New York. ISBN 0-8261-1309-5.

Schaie, K.W. & Pietrucha, M. (Eds.) (2000). Mobility and transportation in the elderly. Springer Publishing, New York. ISBN 0-8261-1309-5.

Spirduso, W.W. (1995). Physical dimensions of aging. Human Kinetics, Champaign, IL, USA. ISBN 0-87322-323-3.

Tacken, M., Marcellini, F., Mollenkopf, H. & Ruoppila, I. (Eds.). (1999). Keeping the elderly mobile. Outdoor mobility of the elderly: problems and solutions. TRAIL Conference Proceedings Series No. P99/1. Delft University Press, Delft.

Transportation Research Board (1998). Transportation in an aging society. Washington D.C.: TRB, special report 218.

Suggested websites

http://www.nationalacademies.org/trb/homepage.nsf
Website of transportation Research Board.

http://www.talkingroads.org
Website providing information on older drivers.

http://www.itsa.org
Website of the international Intelligent Transportation System Information Clearinghouse.

CHAPTER SIX

Information and Communication

Introduction

What do we think of when we use the terms information and communication? Radio, telephones, computers? Each of these categories no longer exists in simple form. They have been extensively exploded so that "radio," even in your automobile, can mean programmable AM/FM/short-wave bands with a continuous play music-seeking cassette player for enjoyment and education and a CD with custom programming of selections. Soon it will include Internet-radio so that local stations all over the world will be available. In addition to auditory input, the possibilities include auditory output–a two-way citizen band transmitter, short-range walkie-talkies and pagers so that we're never out of touch. The word "telephone" now covers mobile phones with memories and roaming capabilities, as well as some things that are just arriving: videophones and world-wide Internet telephony.

The list goes on and on, and is growing. Information and Communication Technologies (ICT) have become so sweeping and pervasive that they underlie nearly all of society's dynamics. For example, worldwide air traffic rests substantially on its communications infrastructure; modern local trade and global competition would be unthinkable without networks of computer servers and effective fiber optics, phone lines and satellites. Even the simple act of driving to work is enhanced by helicopter information about the wrecks and traffic jams ahead. In business, employees in remote places cope with budget cuts and downsizing by utilizing teleconferencing and information from the Internet.

Box 6.1 Use of ICT by older people

Data on the usage of information related equipment as a function of age in The Netherlands.

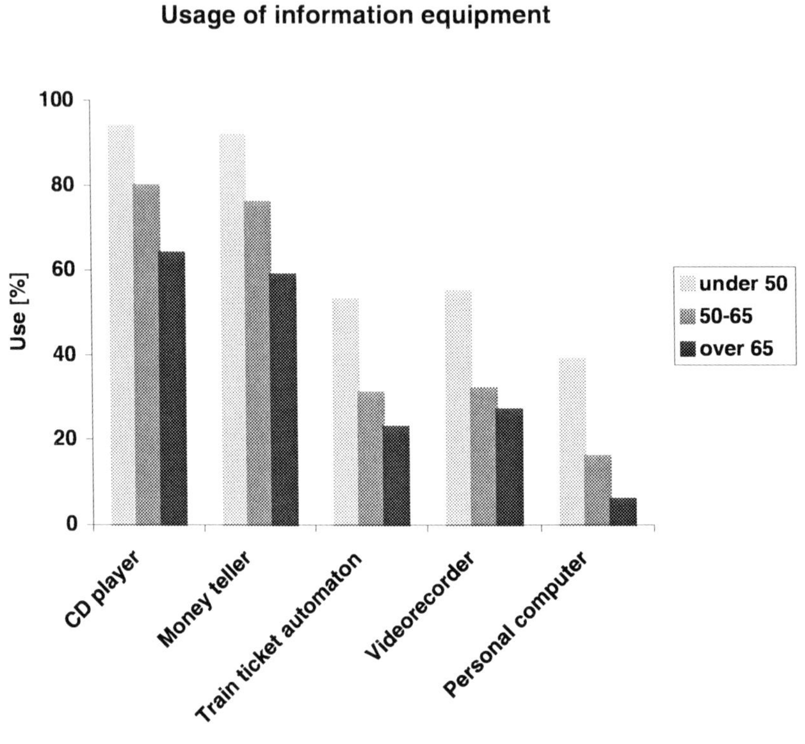

Usage of information equipment
100
80
60
40
20
0
Use [%]
under 50
50-65
over 65
CD player
Money teller
Train ticket automaton
Videorecorder
Personal computer

Figure 1 Usage of information related equipment as a function of age in the Netherlands (Doets & Huisman, 1997). The left three devices are "have ever used," the right two devices are "use regularly."

Doets, C. & Huisman, T. (1997). Digital skills. The state of the art in the Netherlands, CINOP, 's Hertogenbosch, the Netherlands.

Problems with keeping up

In this torrent of technology a person has to have training perpetually and hands-on experience with relevant new products and services. Otherwise it is difficult to participate fully in society. As functionality and complexity of the technologies behind the machines and systems have been increasing, the actual usage has been growing more complex. There are many obvious problems for the older user who is hoping to keep up.

As it was with housing and health and mobility, the problems are highly variable in nature. We need to be careful when generalizing and remember that older individuals have long life histories filled with diverse experiences. Some have technical backgrounds, others don't. They are very heterogeneous as a group, also with respect to information and communication.

Furthermore, we have to remember that the seventy year old of today is qualitatively different from the seventy year old of ten years ago or the seventy year old to come ten years from now, just because of the very rapid pace of the technological changes we have been discussing. The technologies that people are willing and able to use vary widely, obvious when we consider features of telephones, TVs, VCRs, sidewalk money machines, and automatic ticket dispensers.

What is this contraption?

The first problem is that the functionality of devices aren't always recognizable–what can this thing do for me? Why should I buy it or use it? More and more, products and services offer many choices for the user, but often keep their full functionality a secret; for example, personal computers and their programs, VCRs, smart telephones, and many other interfaces to information do this. For instance, most people don't know what all the "function" keys on their computers do even though they may work with the computers daily. Labels such as "F1" and "F2," which stare blankly at us from the PC keyboard are almost totally devoid of meaning.

How do you start and stop it? Click start? Run? End? Halt? Abort? Whoa? Giddyup?

Second, how do you control the device? The challenge of simply making a computer go illustrates the problem. Whoa and giddyup worked well for the machines of the American Old West, horses. Why we didn't preserve continuity here is a puzzle. Click "giddyup" and the machine starts: click "giddyup" and the program starts. "Whoa" stops them both. Then young and old both would understand.

Instead we use terms like "boot," derived from "pulling oneself up by one's bootstraps." These whimsical names are useful in a sense. They make computer terminology more interesting and they stick in human memory better; some are very clever and amusing, but we have to remember them. That's OK, once when we are learning, but then next year we have to remember a new set. Often the new ones are logical only in terms of the previous set, which was whimsically not logically based. Perhaps some standardized set of terms that elude more directly to function needs to be developed. Chemistry has its rules for naming compounds. Young people taking their first course on computers or reading through the manual of their first new computer at Christmas time are willing and eager to memorize whatever is presented simply because of the allure and glitter of the new experience. Older people have already spent much of this "novelty memory." They want to just use the old terms, never mind the amusement– let's get right to the computing.

This is an issue of communication that affects everyone, of course, but the burgeoning technical vocabulary, the morass of borrowed, re-defined, and misshapen words that are appropriated to describe the features of products, especially of computers, creates a special rift for seniors.

The people, mostly young, that name the technology, write the manuals and the labels and instructions and interfaces out there on the frontiers of development speak a different technical language than older people do. Today, the older your knowledge is, the more difficult it is for you to understand these new things. Ironically, even the graduates in computer science itself find themselves "old" in this sense very quickly. The majority of their skill and information can become obsolete in only a couple of years.

The bumble factor

All paths of action that lead to the functionality of a computer or VCR should always be intuitively obvious to all ages. This is never the case, so at least, the user should be able to bumble around and get to the right place eventually. But often the "bumble factor" which at worst should be zero (just bumbling around gets you nowhere) is highly negative. Make the wrong bumble and you can format your hard drive or destroy a month's work, and do it much more easily than you can produce a simple table or graph. Bumbling is based on intuition. "Control-alt Z worked with my word processing program so it should also work here." Such intuitions are based on past experience. The difficulty is that a high bumble factor for an older person with different kinds of experience may imply a low factor for a youth and visa versa. But again, it is the youths that are designing and naming the interfaces.

Just training older people isn't enough, they have to keep on learning

The names of things and functions don't hold still. In the most remote past, we shut down the computer in mid instruction by just turning it off, or by pulling out the plug–no one had trouble remembering this. Later, to stop a program we had to push two keys simultaneously, "control" and "c." Pushing alt break worked for a while but as technology flourished we had to upgrade our skills and learn "control" "alt" "delete," the so called "three finger salute," three keys at once to stop the contraption. Those were the "crude" modern ways of shouting "whoa." Now we have progressed to a new level of sophistication. In one popular operating system the order to STOP the computer is hidden in the START menu! That's right, to stop, you click start.

Box 6.2 Slowed listening

If the rate of speech goes up, then the intelligibility goes down, and this is particularly true when listening conditions are sub-optimal, such as in a noisy environment. Slowing down the speech rate automatically by computer would seem to be a good solution. But the quality of speech usually suffers, and pitches become lower thus affecting the intonation. NHK Science and Laboratories in Tokyo have applied new technology for processing speech that can slow down the rate of speech automatically while maintaining perfect quality including preserving the intonation. The principle rests on repeating of a percentage of full pitch periods of the speech signal, which requires an instantaneous and pitch-synchronous analysis of the speech signal to begin with. Since the principle depends on the properties of the speech signal itself it works for many different languages; in fact, it was first shown to work for French a number of years ago. NHK has also built a microprocessor that does the job on-line and on this basis has developed a consumer device that can be plugged into any ordinary radio or TV appliance.

The increased intelligibility is particularly helpful for listeners with hearing problems and most of these are found among the older people. Since more time is needed for the speech, the system requires pauses in the speech from time to time so that it can catch up, otherwise some portions of the speech can be lost. However, such pauses occur spontaneously and in that case the system can spread the speech out in time, into the pauses, and reproduce all speech in delayed fashion.

Charpentier, F. and Moulines, E. (1989). Pitch-synchronous waveform processing techniques for text-to-speech synthesis using diphones. Eurospeech, 2, 13-19.

Mutsuhashi, T. (1998). Human-friendly broadcasting technology. NHK R&D, 50, 53-59.

Verhelst, W.D.E. (1991). A system for prosodic transplantation with research applications. IPO Annual Progress Report, 26, 29-38.

Walk a mile in their shoes

It is very difficult to put one's self in the position of an older person. Most of us who have come to use forefront technology have, somehow, adapted and forgotten how difficult the learning process was. So it is difficult for us to appreciate all of the reasons a senior might choose to avoid, for example, a computer.

We click start to stop and fumble grudgingly through the obscure menus daily, mercifully unable to recall the agonies of learning and trying to remember.

Pause for a moment to recall the time you've wasted finding and forgetting "paper source" which is for some reason invisible until you bumble into "page setup," which itself is misleadingly hidden in the "files" menu. One can easily think of five or ten similar rat's nests. Recall through the eyes of an older person the time when you tackled the infamous cauldrons of confusion in the pull down menus, "preferences," "options," "advanced," "special" and "set up." Such computing is like untangling a fishing line, brutally demanding for the finest of human memories. You have to open menus one by one to find out where they go, what's in them, what else each item is attached to; and you have to then remember what their ineptly named entries mean from a month ago when you last did this.
If you were an older person without much experience in this realm why would you ever want any? How can we help them to deal with this? How can we make them do anything but want to avoid technology?

Prevention of Problems with Communication

Anything that facilitates or even maintains the process of communication is of potential value to the older persons in this area. They may profit in a number of possible ways. They may be shut in or partially isolated from their friends and families, they may need to replace social links lost to retirement, they may want to reach out electronically instead of physically going to the store or library, and they may need to feel as though emergency communication is always available. So prevention of loss of these things is quite important.

Gerontechnology's focus

Of course, communication may prevent loneliness, isolation, and a host of other obvious problems that concern gerontechnology, and information can provide self-enrichment; but the point here is different. Here we focus on the prevention of problems with communication, per se, rather than on the problems that communication and information can prevent. For instance, the danger of being outdistanced by the technology, completely swamped by it, unable to use it, unable to train for it, unable to fathom it, unable to even obtain it, can perhaps be prevented.

Some devices are almost immediately easy to use for seniors, such as perhaps the videophone. Because they are a simple extension of technology that is for the most part already familiar, older people can be expected to use it with ease. They can show pictures of their grandchildren, exchange engineering diagrams, and enjoy "seeing the kids" more frequently. At the other end of the continuum of usability we find the devices such as the computer, where the seniors are more likely to be left behind.

Electronic prevention of loss–substituting silicon for synapses

More and more, the abrupt distinction between the user and the computers and other interfaces to information is blurring. Much of the intelligence that we users once had to supply is embedded in the interface. Smarter and smarter user interfaces are evolving. We have smart digital assistants, scores of helper programs, hoards of specialized task wizards and other wise digital creatures. We are developing "agents," programs that can handle fragments of our tasks for us, and we can embed these agents, which are not terribly smart individually, into smart configurations with other agents that can deal with more complexity.
We call this "agent architecture." So, more and more, we don't have to be so intelligent personally.

The problem in relation to older persons is mainly one of compatibility. We have to be sure that the seniors and their interfaces understand one another. This means that either the people who develop the interfaces have to remain oriented in part to older people, test the devices on them, let them help with the designs, and so on, or older people have to learn to communicate differently.

Box 6.3 Videophone

The notion of the videophone has been around for some decades. But acceptance has been restricted, both in business and privately. Now that bandwidth limitations are gradually removed both by more efficient coding schemes and by actually increased bandwidth, cheap video telephony has become a real option.

For older persons, this opens up a number of opportunities.
In Europe, some of these have already been tried out and assessed in pilot projects.
A German pilot tried out a cable-tv connection of some 15 older people to a care center, offering remote care-on-demand, counseling, training and service support, and information.
A Finnish pilot provided a videophone service for safety, remote advice, and guidance. Some 40 homes were connected.
A Netherlands pilot used video to assist older hearing-impaired people with lip reading. It also provided medical, social, and informational support such as requests for meals on wheels, pedicures and hairdressers at home, medical help service, shopping support, financial counseling, and a video-telephone circle with other participants of the pilot.
A Portuguese pilot gave support to visually impaired people and those with reduced mobility. It ran a service center in Aveiro with video communications to the users and between the users themselves.

All those pilots thus studied the efficacy of applications in a number of diverse, realistic settings. The various recommendations can now readily be applied for opening a new dimension in prevention. The overall focus of the pilots was on assisting people with special needs, most of which happen to belong to the categories of older people. The pilots also showed that video telephony can be made to be relatively simple and easy to operate by the users, and that subjects generally appeared to enthusiastically accept the new opportunities. Also, it can be expected that video telephony will be cost-effective, since it may save a number of visits of professionals to the older people's homes.

Noorden, L.A. van & McEwan, J. (1992). Pilot applications for advanced communication technology in care for the elderly in Europe.
In: Bouma, H. & Graafmans, J.A. (Eds.). Gerontechnology. IOS Press, Amsterdam. ISBN 90-5199-072-3.

Prevention by training is one answer.

Older people, as a group, are as capable as anyone of dealing with today's bramble bushes of information and communication. But they don't have the same exposure that young people do. How can this be helped?

For one thing, we can replicate the training opportunities that young people get which older people are excluded from. For instance, many people get their first hands-on experiences with some of the new developments in their job situations. For example, people who might not have used a computer at home may be required to use one at work–and trained to do so.
If a person is no longer in the work force this on-going introduction to new devices needs to be sustained in some other way; or other solutions need to be developed.

One solution would incorporate the idea of drop-in centers. Why can't we simulate the portions of the workplace that allow the people at work to learn the new systems? Put fragments of the workplace here and there in the retired person's environment? The fragments would be like "Link Trainers," the early flight simulators, simulating various tasks and systems. These could be perhaps associated with senior centers, perhaps with libraries or courthouses or public parks or universities or other schools or grocery stores for that matter. They would be places where older people could come to learn about the new technology and benefit from it.
Maybe seniors could teach others at these sites.

Accessibility to training, to devices, to instruction and help

There are some studies suggesting that older individuals in a test group of subjects responded differently to challenges in the technological environment than some younger individuals. For instance, they were quicker to walk away from bad interfaces. In some sense, they restricted their own access. The reasons for this are of secondary importance: boredom, mellowness, or fear; the significant fact is that it can happen. They may also restrict their own access by experiencing fewer training opportunities, feeling stupid and blaming themselves rather than the interfaces to technology. Also, older people may tend to have low income limiting their purchasing power and thus their access to classes and equipment.

> ### Box 6.4 Senior net
>
> In the assessment of Hugh O'Connor, Director of AARP's Research Information Center, "The web has the potential to transform the entire experience of aging," coalesces nicely with an October 1998 announcement from Redmond, Washington. "Microsoft to provide computer literacy training to more than 250,000 seniors by the year 2000." One million dollars were granted toward this end to Senior Net. Senior Net is a nonprofit organization providing older adults with education and access to computer technology including the Internet. This is timely action. According to a Department of Commerce study by the National Telecommunications Information Administration of the United States released in July of 1998, less than 10% of seniors are connected to the Internet, and slightly over 20% even own PC's. This is changing rapidly. Senior Net's mission is to connect seniors to the web so that they can share their knowledge with the rest of the world, and of course learn as well, and communicate with friends and relatives and find or work on jobs. The relation between Microsoft and Senior Net thus far has led to the training of 100,000 older adults to use computers and the Internet, to which Microsoft has contributed two million dollars already. In the next year this new grant will allow Senior Net to upgrade the facilities at its 140 learning centers and to add at least 60 more. Half of these will be located in under-served and rural communities.

Prevention of problems by design

Quite a few of the services for information and communication and the devices that have been developed are not adapted to the eyes/ears/minds/fingers of older users. One of our most traditional sources of information, the museum, even spells trouble for the aging eye. The lettering on many exhibits is small, low in contrast, displayed in dim illumination, and placed at a considerable distance behind the glass.

We need to develop and disseminate new techniques of designing for the older person as when we considered the redesign of housing. If a design is good they won't be so inclined to distance themselves from it. But the situation is far from simple.

Countless guidelines have been drawn up for designing nearly every conceivable category of device to be friendly to older people.

There are many charts and diagrams and graphs and tables that characterize the older persons with respect to communication. But there is a sea of tradeoffs that need to be taken into account. For example, consider visual acuity in relation to illumination and magnification in reading.
Older people can read smaller letters if the contrast of the letters with their backgrounds is increased. But a tradeoff is that such a change might be unpleasant and "hard on the eyes" for people who didn't need it, glaring for people with cataracts, and so on. Another way of interpreting this is to say that people can read low-contrast letters, such as most of the LCD screens on personal organizers now present us with, if the letters are made larger. But then fewer lines of text will fit on the screen, which would annoy people who didn't need the increased size.

So still, the problem in the end always is, "What is 'an older person' with respect to this device?" Who is it that I am designing this computer monitor for? Does this person have yellowed lenses or nice plastic implants?
Do they need more contrast, more intensity, less glare, or a purple picture? There is of course no answer because of the vast differences. Let's think our way into the problem a bit. There won't be any final answer, but we'll see some of the scenery of opportunity for gerontechnology.

Obviously, building flexibility into the device that is undergoing design is the only general solution. But there are many forms of flexibility. It doesn't simply mean incorporating a row of buttons for adjusting all of the parameters, which TV sets already have and few people use very much. The knobs interact with one another, they are inconvenient, and it takes time to set them, and so forth.

How about customization to the individual viewer? But simply developing presets so that Viewer 'A' can adjust the buttons and call all of the settings back at any time by pushing 'A' may not work either.
For one thing, different people who like different presets may be viewing the monitor simultaneously.

How about having every person carry his or her own monitor around? They can adjust it the way they want to and keep it that way all of the time. Too heavy? Not anymore. There are viewing devices under development that will fit in your pocket. A miniature monitor that fits on your glasses is in the immediate technological future.

The image will fill your visual field, not just the few millimeters of retina that video monitors now stimulate. It will be in visual stereo too.

So, the problem of older people using monitors is solved? Not yet. It would be very easy to accidentally exclude older people by virtue of design, simply because they can't accommodate the lenses in their eyes to change focus–or for a hundred other reasons. Industry could easily spend a lot of money in research and design and get locked into the production of a device that the general public loved that older people wouldn't ever use because of the glare, the misfocus, the eye strain, and so on. Encouraging conformance to visual systems of older people, and testing with older populations, among the designers is one function we can't neglect.

Take hearing difficulties as an example. In many, if not all, older people the hearing threshold is raised, starting with the highest frequencies and gradually reaching out toward the lower frequencies where speech sounds reside. But for males the effects are stronger than for females perhaps because of different working environments. Figure 1.2 provides average results, which of course should not be confused with the very heterogeneous results of individual males or females. Interestingly, visual difficulties are generally more prominent in females.

As an additional nicety, an offshoot of prevention, could we encourage the developers of this or any other product to try and solve some other problems that could relate to the older people at the same time? What comes to mind in terms of finding some such device–a super smart interface to the retinas that can display just about anything?
A magnifier/telescope, all books in one, a purveyor of any information you can think of? What other uses might there be?

Prevention by creative complaining about design

Seniors aside, our interfaces with information and communication, and our devices, will have to be modified anyway, for the sake of all of us. We all dislike them and moan about them constantly, so in order to sell more units and compete with one another, the companies will have to eventually begin to worry. Thus, one important function of gerontechnology here is in complaining loudly from the older persons' point of view. The clamor should be senior-oriented: about keyboards that are too stiff for older people, displays that are too dim, double clicks that come too fast, systems that are unnecessarily complex, systems that have generational barriers, systems that deliver products too oriented to youth, systems that bore older people or that are too slow or too fast or too unfamiliar for them.

Be imaginative

Again, we need your originality as well as your intolerance. We ask you to abandon your preconceptions about communication and information.
We have adapted to a number of problems to the extent that we don't even see them as problems anymore. The older people have too–it doesn't occur to anyone to complain. Remember that the common keyboard we center many of our thoughts about interfacing with information on, which we have become so used to and have so innocently invested thousands of hours learning to use, was deliberately designed, according to rumor anyhow, to frustrate us, to be very slow so that we users wouldn't out-type the first primitive typewriters and embarrass the inventor. Yet, we continue to put up with such things not ever realizing how mad we should be.
The older people do too.

Similarly, keep in mind that the design of interfaces is still wallowing in various analogs of primitive flat 2-dimensional paper–"pages," screens of information, windows and the like, layered occasionally, but totally static in the third dimension, unlike most rich sources of information that people are used to in the real world. We should be zooming through dynamic three-dimensional corridors and forests of information like Luke Skywalker, not hobbling from screen to screen and from menu item to puzzling menu item. Most of our natural experiences aren't so restricted and our thoughts about design shouldn't be either. Think for a moment about the comprehensiveness of our interfaces. For instance, if we have a remote control that only can control the television, and another that controls the garage door, and one that controls the VCR, and one that locks the doors of the house and the car, and so on, isn't that too many remotes and control devices? Can we do it all with one? A personal super-key that makes the whole world of a person's technology go and stop and change and open and close. But if we personally have trouble with the VCR's remote and also with the TV's remote, won't we be completely swamped by the two-in-one box? Won't older people be? Not if we design with their human perceptual, cognitive, and motor parameters well in mind.

And if we do, other users, still younger, may love to use these as well. Then, this can be rightly called, "Design for all."

Also, as we did before, let's dissect–each individual need or desire, on close scrutiny, may emerge as being composed of many separate components, each of which can be satisfied separately, and simply. Developers may not choose to do this without some gerontechnological goading from us. And remember a specific desire may dissect into different components for young and old in several ways. The requirements for information and communications, the desired results, the necessary leverages on the world, are all different.

Imagine how an effective ideal personal digital assistant (PDA) serving as an intellectual and informational prosthetic might look like. PDAs are being designed to turn normal people into super intellects with hand-held memory with more and more impressive functionality. Is there any reason older people who are declining mentally can't still join in and be super too? Yes, mis-design of the interface and lack of flexibility in function.

Compensation

Compensation in the areas of information and communication might be best exemplified by the compensation for lost functioning that computers are becoming so good at. For instance, if the demands of dealing with a screen become too much, a person can switch to an auditory output so that the message that used to appear on the screen is now spoken, and the loss is compensated for. Typing can be replaced by voice recognition, devices for controlling the cursor such as mouses, joy sticks, scratch pads, digitizing tablets, and touch screens can be interchanged with one another to compensate for difficulties with elbow movement that the mouse requires, difficulty with wrist movement that the joystick may demand, difficulty with controlling a single finger on the scratch pad, the difficulty with holding the stylus of the digitizing tablet, or the shoulder movements involved in operating a touch screen or an air mouse. In each case, the same goal, pointing, is achieved by compensating for the loss of mobility that is peculiar to the pointing task in some way.

Box 6.5 Warning signals

In earlier technological times the main alarm signals in the home were the doorbell and later the bell of the telephone. Sounds such as these cover wide frequency spectra and are distinguishable in various ways, partly because of their different time courses. The phone rings repeatedly. Also it may have a different sound than the doorbell. Nowadays, many of the appliances in the house have built in alarms, making it necessary for a person to differentiate between different sounds to determine what a given alarm signal is all about.

With their deficits in the higher frequencies, older people have more trouble making these discriminations. They may also have trouble even hearing the higher alarms, such as are produced by pocket organizers and wrist watches. Older people need more intensity to hear those high frequencies, especially in noisy environments. But intensity means energy, which may be in scarce supply in a small device such as a watch. However, technology can supply alarms with adjustable characteristics that people can adjust to match their own personal characteristics. Or alarms can be made adaptive. For example, when in noisy environments smart alarms could automatically increase intensity or alter their sounds or modes (perhaps buzzing the skin) in order to identify themselves better.

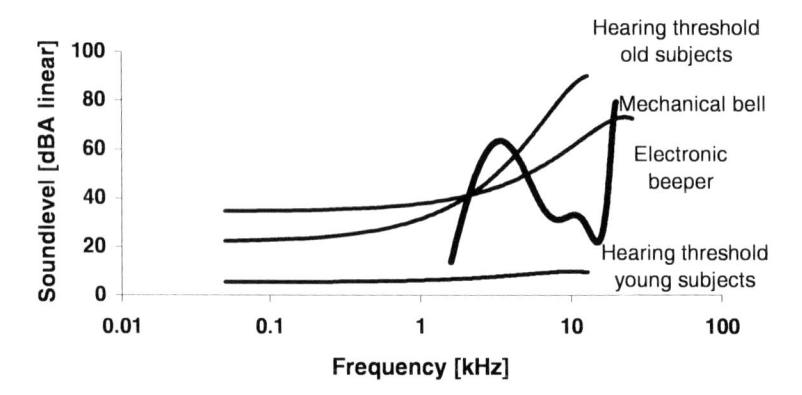

Figure 1 Schematic sound spectra of beeper and mechanical bell as compared to average hearing thresholds of young and old subjects.

> Moving toward present times, the spectrum of the electronic beeper is characteristically and anathema for older people with hearing loss. First, because they are usually small, residing in tiny areas such as in watches, and are designed to save energy and may be driven by a Quartz crystal with low mechanical power, they are very quiet in the lower frequency ranges where older people hear more effectively. Of course, the intensity of such a device can be increased so that it is above threshold. But, doing this can easily exceed what is known as the "terminal threshold" in hearing–the point where pain sets in. The ears of older people are more sensitive in this way and a shrill sound can be rather painful.
>
> Also, as we note elsewhere, high frequency sounds are more difficult to localize. This would explain the older person who hears someone's wrist alarm going off but doesn't realize that it is his own. This latter concern applies more strongly to signals such as smoke detectors, microwave ovens, stoves which are loud enough to be heard but may be more difficult to localize and that may all sound nearly the same since they may be based on essentially the same physical device.
>
> Research is needed into ways to break through the hearing barriers by crafting timbres that can both be heard and can be distinguished from one another from device to device.
>
> Kuchinomachi, Y. et al. (1997). The relationship between the usability of daily electric appliances and the deterioration in cognitive function of old people. Proceedings of the 13th triennial Congress of the International Ergonomic Association. 5, 591-593.

Leliveld & Waterham (1992) discuss early discoveries of applications of aids in communication for the older persons through voice synthesis and recognition in gerontechnology. Several applications for the handicapped and older persons have been realized that can lessen the difficulties with computer interfaces. There is an imminent explosion of devices that convert text to speech, and speech to text. Speech can range from single words from a restricted vocabulary up to full sentences in unrestricted vocabulary. Progress in this field of endeavor is steady and will change the user interface in the coming years, not only for people with specific handicaps, but for everybody. Compensation in this sense is a matter of remapping functionality of one sort onto functionality of another. Sometimes the remapping is obvious. If you can't see the information, maybe you can still feel it, as is the case with Braille. Or, the information that is being missed because of diminished vision can be changed into auditory information as is done with clicking "walk" signals at intersections.

Suppose you wanted to remap the visual information on a computer screen bursting with information from the Internet complete with colors, icons, text and movement, onto a tactile pad, or onto the auditory system as a field of sounds. Is it possible? How might one accommodate the sensibilities of the older people? The information on the screen can be dissected, in millions of useful ways, and various replacement candidates can be chosen by trial and error. To illustrate, color running through the spectrum from violet to red on the screen could be felt as tactile texture running from smooth to rough on the pad and be heard as timbre running from the smoothness of the flute to the roughness of the bassoon. Or color might be remapped into the frequency of tactile vibration, and the pitches, low to high, of tones.

Alternately, there may be perceptual overload with information coming in all forms to a number of sensory channels, as when a driver is overloaded by signs, rearview mirror, other cars, and the rest of the milieu of traffic. In a major sense, all of the devices from assistive technology that might be used to compensate for some function of hearing or vision or perception should be included in the list of potential gerontechnological solutions.

Enhancement–an example

Communication and information are excellent sources for enhancement. For instance, if older persons want to enhance a drooping life they might develop new horizons by joining a group. In the past, apart from conference calls on the telephone perhaps, joining a group meant that each member had to travel to where the group was to meet. With the power of Internet-like entities for communication this is no longer necessary.
Let's think through a simple example to see how it might go. As it was with the smart toilet and other supertech systems that may exist in the future, these hypothetical systems that we conjure up here aren't necessarily important in their own right, nor necessarily even feasible nor attainable. That doesn't matter here because they only need to serve as

organizing frameworks for our thoughts about general principles in the application of technology. They facilitate thought and communication. If we can assemble the ideas and technology, even if only mentally or on paper, that would allow one kind of distributed social group to exist for the older persons, then we can do it for many others.

We will be thinking about group painting for the next few paragraphs. Possibly you would like to think in parallel about applying the same approach to some different group activity–maybe your hypothetical senior would prefer to play the trombone in a "world wide web distributed" Dixieland band of the future or collaborate in designing a new circuit or simply share an activity with one other person.

The activity of group painting offers us a window into distributed social group activities in general, where the participants are in different locations. There are several interesting questions that we can only guess about. Can the experience be as gratifying and educational as the "real" thing, or do you really have to travel to a meeting with real people to be gratified? It's better, in some ways, to go to a concert personally rather than watch it on TV, but with group painting we have a very different situation. The tele-group is interactive–you are one of the performers. Is there anything in the experience that will be missing? Is there anything we can add to the electronic experience that the real thing might be missing? Fascinating questions.

Let's think big according to the rule: if you can think of a need in gerontechnology, we can eventually find the technology for it. Our initial equipment list includes a couple of video cameras for each senior's studio, one pointing at the senior and the easel, one covering the canvas so that every person will be able to see all of the other people's paintings. We'll need a super ISDN line to eliminate annoying delays as you upload and download all of this video information in real time.

Oh yes, some oils and brushes and a canvas; unless you would prefer to design this system totally around the computer, in terms of one of the big graphics painting programs, maybe Corel Photo Paint, and forget the brushes and other messy things altogether. Then many personal problems with motor control and sensory aberration can be eliminated. For instance, in the case of tremor we can filter out those tremor frequencies

electronically from the "brush" so that the trembling person can paint with complete steadiness. Aberrations in color vision can be offset too.
We can enhance the violet colors for the older person who doesn't see them as strongly, so that the finished picture won't look violet to everyone else.

It's awfully quiet, we forgot the microphones–it's no fun at such a gathering unless everyone can converse. (But now you can turn the loud people down without their knowing about it.)

We need to focus some cameras on the model. A given artist won't be able to zoom a given camera because that would bother the other artists, but the individual artist can zoom his/her own screen at will to "walk up close" or "stand back," and can switch to different views of the model. A person can "move back" from one's own work by looking through a camera in the room that is pointed at it and zoomed back. This would be handy for everyone and essential for some handicapped.

The only thing remaining is the control interface to switch between the various views–the whole room view, the views of the individual paintings, the views of the painters, and so on. It too can be designed so that there is customized enhancement, it can be voice controlled, saying a person's name brings up their image maybe. In a real setting such as this it would be wise to sit behind the best artist in the group and learn by copying brush strokes, layout, shading, coloration, and ideas. But here, you can sit behind everybody, one at a time of course, by just switching between cameras. And each of the people can sit behind you and copy your ideas too, make helpful suggestions about your layout perhaps–but you can block your own camera if you don't want that to happen; at first while you're just learning, point it at a Rembrandt.

If this is done right, it should give the impression of being in a real group, the people can talk to each other, "move" around by switching cameras, see each other's work, look at each other and so on. Of course the possibilities are endless–this could be a Christmas gathering, or a cooking club, collaboration on a book, an engineering class, a choir, a reading of fairy stories to the distributed grandchildren, a piano lesson for one of them, a barbershop quartet, a jam session, a chamber ensemble, a group lesson in foreign language, each of course with different problems of implementation, but the technology is available.

At the extreme sometimes we may need to worry about too much technology of interaction, more than some people might want.
For example, consider a physiological/psychological total home page. It might include all of the things that we could possibly monitor embedded in the home page. Among other things, such a possibility brings up the question of when technology is intrusive. As we do with our personalities, we probably want to distribute our personal information onto several home pages selectively depending on whom they are intended for. Many people, especially the very old, might like to have their doctor privy to all of the physiological part of their homepages, perhaps in case of emergency, perhaps just for the comfort of being monitored. Many people however would not want their friends to have constant access to their physiology, but might give them the "feelings" part of the page, the financial section might be more secret, recent personal news could go either way. A person's conglomeration of home pages will be similar to the rooms in one's house, especially as they become visually and auditory three-dimensional and come to resemble rooms rather than "pages."

Care assist

In the section on prevention we chose to focus only on deficits of communication and information that can be prevented, not on the problems of older people that communication and information can prevent.
In this section we turn to look at the importance of communication and information itself in caring for older people.

In the days gone by on the frontiers, in the days when we diagnosed our own illnesses, rode to the doctor on a horse and recovered alone at home, the primary burden of awareness, of care and responsibility fell on us as individuals. Now, once the sound of the siren or the slap of the rotors is heard, our responsibility pretty much is over. The team hooks us up to tubes and electrodes, transports us and we recover as some gentle caring computer watches our every breath and heartbeat with great wisdom and concern. Communication of information makes this and other more advanced scenarios possible for thousands of people every day.

Givers of care are facing astounding new leverage from advances in communication and information. This technology is bringing us to a time when 24-hour private nursing and response to crisis will be common, although some of this nursing will stem from silicon in the form of computerized analysis and services. Some people on the web have already gone so far as to position cameras about in their lives so that the whole world can tune in on their present realities as they live day to day.

But, the technology of communicating sounds and visual images represents only a small fraction of the information that providers of care potentially have access to. Electrocardiograms (EKG), electromyograms (EMG) and the results of ongoing physiological tests even today are routinely sent over the telephone. However, now we have to plan for even more physiological closeness. With smaller and less expensive monitors, coupled with the portability of mobile phones, it will be possible not only for a person who may be feeling faint, for instance, at a given moment to check in to a central diagnostic center to see what's going wrong physiologically.
If one of the big data forecasting programs is tied in at the other end of the line, the providers of care will even see how the person will be in the future, will know how to respond and what advice to give to the person. "You are in insulin shock. Your blood pressure has dropped slightly– please, sit down while testing continues and the global positioning system is accessed." This could be life saving for a cardiac patient or a diabetic. The cumbersome rarely implemented use of a tape recording heart monitor with periodic transmitting of cardiac 'episodes' over the phone lines, and many of the other things that presently are used to diagnose medical problems only after very ominous signs of them arise will soon be things from the distant past.

As we noted previously with respect to home page interfaces to people, there is immense potential for shredding our privacies. In the area of care with all of the additional medical issues the potential for unwanted invasion is even larger. Some older people may want to be totally known to the world or at least to selected friends or relatives. Others such as the heart patients may want only selected parts of their personal information to be available on web pages that can only be accessed by selected individuals, such as their physicians. Most old people may not want to have anything to do with programs of "hyper care," and gerontechnology is careful to respect that: our job is to simply be sure that all the options are there for people to choose from.

Research

The development of communications interfaces for seniors

Computers are moving from the desktop and the palmtop to the wrist and even now some are inside the person. Body nets already exist that transmit information through the skin to distributed computers dispersed on the body. Soon all of these pieces will be able to be hooked together from the informational point of view through segments of the World Wide Web or in other ways. One of our main challenges resulting from these expanding technologies of communication and information is in extrapolating the many emerging possibilities, such as those epitomized by the hypothetical WWW painting group we considered previously. Then we need to conceive of, design, and implement interfaces to the new systems with older people in mind.

As we have noted, seniors may require different interfaces to information and the technology of communicating it. These differences are often important, and they become extremely so when tasks such as driving are considered. For example, Pauzié & Letisserand (1992) point out that the development of sophisticated in-vehicle systems will have the potential for transmitting and hopefully communicating much more information to the driver than we get now. So there is less and less latitude with respect to the formulation, display, and positioning of information because there may be too much of it. To illustrate, these scientists note some characteristics of the display's legibility that may, or may not, be serious problems for seniors depending on the person. We list them here and invite you to provide some of the auditory, cutaneous or proprioceptive parallels.

- Foveal vision with a proper placement of the display in the driver's visual field
- Visual acuity with visual display verbal/symbolic legibility requirements and importance of letter/symbol size, style and contrast
- Visual accommodation and adaptation are critical parameters because drivers are constantly shifting gaze between the instruments and visual targets outside.

Box 6.6 Signal-to-noise ratio of speech

The influence of age on our auditory sensibility is commonly expressed as simply an increase in thresholds for hearing as a function of frequency, presbyacusia. The higher frequencies of sound, typically, become more and more difficult to hear at low levels. Less known, but sometimes even more important, is an elevation of the required signal-to-noise (S/N) ratio. Older people have more difficulty hearing "signals" such as speech or warnings in noisy environments. In fact, a small loss of a few decibels of sensitivity may be quite impairing. Many situations in everyday life happen to be noisy, for example, social happenings, intersections of streets, and public and private transport. Many situations are deliberately loaded with extraneous auditory information, for example with music, that hinder the perception of speech. Unfortunately, amplification with a hearing aid amplifies the noise as well as the signal and leaves the S/N ratio unaffected, so a single hearing aid may not be helpful in this case.

The best remedy is to decrease the level of the interfering noise, but if that isn't feasible, some options are: a smaller distance between the speaker and the listener; use of hearing aids in both ears to provide a sense of localization of the signal in relation to the noise; a microphone that is placed close to the person who is speaking. One can see persons unconsciously attempting to compensate for low S/N ratios in ways that could be translated into technology. They cup their hands around one, or both, ears which deflects some of the noise that isn't coming from the direction of the speaker, just as they improve S/N in conditions of glare by cupping the hands around the eyes. Recall a previous technology that addressed S/N in the same way by shielding out the noise, the cumbersome "ear horn." They turn their heads side ways so that the sound of the speaker's voice comes more directly into the best ear. (This tendency is sometimes used by "mind readers" on stage to mysteriously divine that certain members of the audience have, "some minor medical problem–perhaps something to do with hearing.") And they move their heads closer to give the signal, the speaker's voice, a bit more advantage over the ambient noise of the environment which remains at the same level when they move.

When arrays of factors such as these are coupled with highly demanding situations, the difficulties begin to cascade exponentially.

Too much visual information decreases the signal-to-noise ratio and so sorting out the signal from the noise, the desired information from the useless information, becomes more difficult and sometimes impossible for the brain. This problem extends into all of the modalities.

If you spend a moment thinking about your own car a dozen problems with its interface to you will come to mind that could be more severe for some older persons–and that could perhaps be fixed easily with only minimal research.

Much research is presently being put into the design of smart interfaces. Consider some interesting technological questions remaining. Should the car know that you are presently working to tune the radio or that your attention is otherwise engaged? Should it revise its strategies then for providing other information to you? Should it warn you audibly under certain circumstances of condition-specific things; for instance apprise you of traffic lights and stop signs, but only when it knows you aren't looking at the road? Should the formatting of the information be dependent on circumstances? What circumstances? Could the controls, such as the turn indicator wand, perform different operations under different conditions? Should the car understand your voice? What will happen if a voice on the radio accidentally tells the car to do something dangerous, will the car know and let you compensate in time? Will any of this confuse some people? Who? Most important for us, will these advances be designed so that they help seniors or harm them?

Suggested readings

Bouma, H. (1998). Gerontechnology: Emerging technologies and their impact on aging in society. In: J. Graafmans, V. Taipale & N. Charness. (Eds.). Gerontechnology: A sustainable investment in the future. (pp. 93-104). IOS Press, Amsterdam. ISBN 90-5199-367-6.

Bouma, H. (in press). Document and user interface design for older citizens. In: P.H. Westendorp, C.J.M. Jansen & R. Punselie. (Eds.). Interface Design and Document Design. Rodopi Press, Amsterdam/Atlanta.

Bouwhuis, D.G. (1992). Aging, perceptual and cognitive functioning and interactive equipment. In: H. Bouma & J.A.M. Graafmans. (Eds.), Gerontechnology. Proceedings of the first International Conference on Gerontechnology, Eindhoven, August 1991. (pp. 93-112). IOS Press, Amsterdam. ISBN 90-5199-072-3.

Masthoff, J.F. (1997). An agent-based instruction system. Ph.D dissertation. Eindhoven University of Technology.

Norman, D.A. (1988). The psychology of everyday things. Basic Books, New York. ISBN 0-465-06709-3.

Norman, D.A. (1993). Things that make us smart: Defending human attributes in the age of the machine. Addison-Wesley, New York. ISBN 0-201-58129-9.

Stewart, T. (1992). Physical interfaces or "obviously it's for the elderly, it's grey, boring and dull." In: H. Bouma & J.A.M. Graafmans (Eds.). Gerontechnology. Proceedings of the first International Conference on Gerontechnology, Eindhoven, August 1991. (pp. 197-207). IOS Press, Amsterdam. ISBN 90-5199-072-3.

Suggested websites:

http://www.w3.org/WAI/
Website of the Web Accessibility Initiative.

http://www.cordis.lu/ist/home.html
Website of the EU Information Society Technologies Program: promoting a user-friendly information society.

CHAPTER SEVEN
Mathematical Modeling and Simulation

Introduction

What is a model?

There are many ways to represent objects and processes in the world. We do it physically by painting or drawing pictures of people and nature, we do it in three dimensions with model railroads and dolls. A model might be a drawing, perhaps to scale, of a house with flat paper furniture that we move around to see where it looks nicest and functions best: this is much easier than moving the actual furniture. A model always is easier or better in some way than the real thing. It is lighter, or smaller, or simpler and cheaper to make, or can be tested and destroyed without negative consequences.

What can models do?

Extrapolating these ideas into the realm of gerontechnology, we find that models have far-reaching potential. They give us a microscopic window into the inner chemical worlds of people, for example, we can look at the effects of subtleties of what people eat, whether they exercise, and so on. Or, we can model the way older people walk or drive. We can even model the process of aging itself with respect to lifestyle and the underlying biochemistry and can try out ways of slowing or stopping aging altogether.

A model can do things that the original object can't

Models are usually expendable, flexible, and comprehensive. We can "crash" models of people to see how older people might be damaged in accidents. We can overload them with forces or information to see what the consequences are in specific situations. We might speed them up and watch a lifetime of biochemical change, perhaps in all of the individual digestive processes at once, flow through the various organs in a few seconds.

Then we can do it again under different hypothetical circumstances, maybe with different diet, and see what difference over the lifetime that makes. We can slow some models down, and watch picosecond chemical metabolic reactions spread out in time as free radicals munch away at molecules. We can test models destructively, and perform "unethical" experiments on them. We heat them, cool them, poison them and strain them to see how a human system might behave under similar circumstances.

What can we model?

Models can be models of any aspects of people, of their actions, of their processes of aging, of their reactions to stairs and sidewalks and objects or processes. We can include environmental factors, special tasks that people might be performing, and all of the interactions between these. Models are simply partial analogs: this means that some aspect of the model behaves more or less like some aspect of the thing that is being modeled.

The roles of the gerontechnologist

We can borrow models

First, models already exist that have succeeded impressively in many fields and many of these can be applied directly to various problems of older people. It may seem odd at first thought that the model of the dynamics of a ten-mile antenna floating in space or of a nuclear power plant are of the same form as a model that might be employed to predict when an older person is about to fall down or experience some threatening difficulty with digestion, but it is true. When an applicable model exists already, the gerontechnologist may serve as a go between, talking with scientists and engineers about the possibilities of applying the model to specific problems of the aged.

Alternately, the gerontechnologist who is mathematically trained can be the one who transplants models from other fields, modifying and refurbishing them, and tuning them up for use with older people.

We also may build models

If models that fit the situations and people in question don't exist, then someone with a flare for gerontechnology is needed to clarify the problem to be modeled for the appropriate experts from mathematics, science, or engineering so that they can build the model. Or we can build them ourselves.

Simulation

Mathematical models, to be discussed later, require a mathematician and possibly a great deal of work and time. There are other classes of models, we will call them physical simulations here that can be developed and used in the field with no training in mathematics. Once developed, simulations can be used to generate data about aging that can either be experienced first hand, or can in turn be used in mathematical modeling.

At one end of the continuum, the space agencies, using mathematics and equipment from the frontiers of science, simulate aircraft and space capsules so that astronauts can get experience in them without endangering themselves or the equipment.

In gerontechnology we need the same level of simulation for a number of applications. Most of these are still in the future. However, there are some simpler approaches that we are working on now. For example, we can simulate systems such as bank machines and ticket machines and a host of other tasks so that older people who are not familiar with them can gain experience. We can modify driving and flight simulators to measure performance and to retrain older people. And, we can even simulate aging itself, so individuals associated with aged people, such as designers, family members, scientists, and others can feel what it's like to age. Let us consider a few actual physical simulations for the study of aging.

Box 7.1 Advantages of modeling

- Simplification. Models provide manageable analogs of processes related to aging that are too complex to be dealt with rationally by the human mind.
- Precision.
- Formalization of situations, questions, answers, and issues.
- Organizational frameworks for experimental results.
- Synchronization of interdisciplinary research on problems in the broad field of gerontechnology.
- A language of description and a bridge to other languages, e.g. those of design, physics, safety, engineering, psychology, sociology, chemistry, nutrition, or medicine.
- Prediction of emerging states and events, states of aging, environmental conditions such as indoor climate, accidents such as falling, or illness.
- Data collection that can lead to improved control of aging and its associated processes.
- Short-term monitoring, e.g. of ambulation or attention and comparisons over time.
- Long-term monitoring, e.g. of memory capacity, conglomerates of medical data, or physical and mental condition.
- Development of multidimensional criteria, e.g. for fitness to perform specific functions at work or at home or on the highway.
- Precise design specifications and criteria for safety, comfort, or livability.
- Expert systems specific to the decision-making problems of the gerontechnologist and related practitioners.
- Medical or situational diagnosis and treatment related assistance.
- Links to other models that may all be combined into powerful expert systems that will eventually provide intelligent advise on virtually all of the problems of aging.
- Political leverage. Whereas re-teaching an older person to walk or do arithmetic may not fit into the formalization or the funding structures of academia, mathematical modeling of these processes, or of nearly any other gerontechnological process, probably will.

The simulation of aged ambulation

Ambulation and postural stability become very important in old age. One falls more readily, recovers with less facility, and is damaged more extensively if the recovery fails. As we have noted elsewhere, the sensory inputs from the sole of the foot diminish, the vestibular systems become less functional or worse they generate illusory perceptions of self motion and disorientation, there are visual distortions from bifocals and from other sources in the eye and nervous system, the righting reactions are slower if a fall begins, the gait is more shuffling leading to greater hazard from tripping, the periphery of the visual field narrows and contrast dims sometimes disallowing the perception of trip hazards, and so on. Informative as they might be, these are only words. What is it really like to operate under such conditions?

An actual experiment

Recently, at the University campus, seemingly tipsy young students were seen hobbling about with uncertain gait, tipping to the left and right, and making erratic head movements apparently unable to see normally. Brain damage? No, this was an experiment in the simulation of aging being conducted in a laboratory of the Institute for Gerontechnology. It was found, by comparing the data from artificially impaired students with data from actual older people to validate the simulation, that it is possible to allow a younger person to experience the losses of joint mobility and sensory input that some older people experience (Harrington et al., 1998). In essence, these experimental subjects had been hobbled with knee braces, partially blinded with special glasses, and deprived of both cutaneous sensibility and stable footing by a carpet made from sponge. (Older people often use spongy insoles that deprive them of firm footing and appropriate tactile feedback.)

There were several reasons why this was being done. First, it allowed individuals who didn't have the joint immobility to experience it and report on it. This is useful in both teaching gerontechnology and in studying the ambulation of older people: the student can actually be put into the same situations that older people experience rather than just being told about them. The experimenter can observe what happens without having to jeopardize an older person who might not be able to maintain stability.

Second, this method provides an excellent way of designing for older people who have specific parameters of movement. The designer can simply climb the stairs with the same degree of joint immobility that the older person would have and adjust the stair accordingly, realizing of course that he/she can catch hold etc. better than an aged person in the event of a fall. A younger person in an age simulator may unknowingly proceed with more abandon and have less real cause for concern than a frangible older person might have.

Third, an experiment such as this can be used to collect data for a mathematical model, which can be used to study ambulation, make predictions about when a person is about to fall down and so forth.

The simulation of tremor

Some older people become less steady and tremble for a number of possible neurological reasons. What is the effect of tremor on motor performance? How does it affect the performance of complex tasks such as sewing, or simple tasks such as turning pages? Is it ever dangerous, can you drop things or click the wrong buttons with your mouse because of it? Are there ways to fix it with weights or styles of performing or training?

As you can imagine, there would be a number of problems if one were to try to answer these questions by performing experiments on older people who actually do tremble. The answer instead? Simply devise a simulation of tremor, validate it so that you know the young person is performing just like the older person who trembles would on the task at hand, and measure performance under the various conditions that are of interest–driving, dialing a telephone, picking up a glass at a formal dinner, and so forth.

At the Institute for Gerontechnology, researchers have devised a number of simulations of tremor and a number of representative tasks. For example, a slowly pulsing vibrator is attached to the wrist and the experimental subject is required to turn the pages of a book, thread a needle, spoon liquid. These are normally simple tasks; does tremor defined in this way present any problems? As one might expect, the simulations have led to some discoveries. For example, it had been thought that tremor would manifest itself as purely a motor disturbance. However, it was discovered that in a task such as turning pages an important effect comes about because of the disruption of sensory input that the trembling causes–turning a page requires very fine cutaneous discriminations, which the vibration disrupts.

In another phase of the experiment the cursor on a computer screen is made to tremble as the subject performs a series of pointing tasks. This experiment allows examination of the contribution of the hand-eye components, without the complications of actual hand movement. It also allows the collection of precise mathematical data that is in a perfect form for mathematical modeling. For example, in a tracking task, devised in collaboration with scientists at the Kiev Polytechnic Institute, Peter and Alex Bidyuk, the subject follows a moving target on the computer screen using the mouse as a pointing device. The computer, in addition to moving the target and making the cursor tremble, watches the difference in their respective positions very closely and records every detail. At the end of the trial the computer calculates parameters of performance, such as the mean square error, the frequency response of the person, and so on, and stores these with the moment to moment data–perfect for the mathematical modeler who may want to characterize older people in terms of such performance, or may want to generalize the performance to other tasks.

The need for other simulations of aging: Shade tree psychophysics

Rather than deal with complex laboratory equipment in a complex experimental setting that may well produce data that doesn't transform to actual application, it may be easier to simply jury rig a simulation, quick but adequate, much like the "shade tree mechanic" works on cars.

Perhaps you yourself would like to devise and try out some type of simulator to reproduce some of the possible effects of aging with respect to some task? Reaction time can be slowed in a simulation by dimming the stimulus. Response time can be increased with large rubber bands and effective strength can be lessened elastically or with weights. Devices for simulating joint pain, perhaps using a strain gauge and a device for shocking electrically are easy to contrive and can be quite educational when trying to screw the lid from a jar or when performing other motor activities. In fact, nearly every aspect of ambulating with an aging motor system can be simulated.

Simulating aging with a wedge

Simulations of aging sensory systems are also possible. One way of accomplishing this is with one of the many types of "wedge." For example, there is some dimming of vision with age. In photography a neutral density filter dims the image, as do sun glasses. The problem is getting the "model," the filter, adjusted so that a normal viewer sees the same amount of dimming as a specific older person–they are all different. The solution is a neutral density wedge. This is a strip of photographic film that progresses smoothly from being completely clear at one end to being completely dark at the other. In between it dims the vision to varying degrees when the observer looks through it.

This is letter size wedge

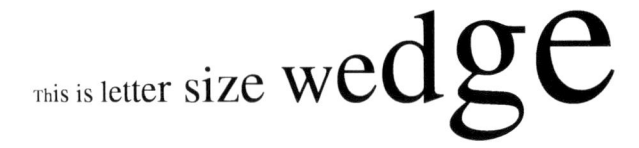

Figure 7.1 Letter size wedge

One can construct a wedge for letter size. To use the letter size wedge, one can have the subject view the wedge from the specific viewing distance, on the monitor screen, down the hall etc. Ask them to indicate the smallest letter or word they can easily read under these conditions. Then put yourself in their optical shoes: For instance, if they indicate the "s" in the word "size" is unreadable at one meter, back away until you also can barely make out that letter. This will give you a way in a sense to see through their eyes when viewing in other circumstances–just back away that same proportionate distance and look at the scene. Then you can enlarge the letter size etc. so you are comfortable with it at that distance, and then they may also be able to read it from their normal viewing distance. Be sure to test whether this is really true in the given case. There are a number of other factors involved such as accommodation, glare, and the rest of the visual mechanics.

To calibrate one's vision in terms of contrast to that of some older person in a specific situation, say reading, lay a density wedge on the text of interest. The text will be easily readable through the clear end of the filter, unreadable at the dark end, and barely readable somewhere in between. The older person will probably see the "unreadable" point as being considerably more toward the light end of the filter than someone younger will, especially if there is glare from a light source that is near the line of sight. If the younger person slides the filter until the same text that the older person noted was barely visible becomes barely visible, and marks the point, then later, under similar conditions of viewing, the younger person can simply look through the filter at that same point and know whether similar text would be readable by that specific older person.

A number of other sensory wedges are possible that could be used in gerontechnology and need to be devised and validated by actual experimentation. The size wedge, similar to the eye chart of the optician, of course would have letters that become smaller and smaller as we have seen.

The glare wedge simulates the progressive lack of transparency of the lens of the eye as people age. The effect is that of a dirty windshield when one is driving into the sun. An older person "sees" the lens in the eye itself because of light bouncing from it, and within it, more than a younger person, and can't see beyond these illuminated surfaces. To make a glare wedge you can put down semi-overlapping layers of thin plastic, such as some plastic sheet protectors like the ones we keep our important papers sheathed in.

One can make a color wedge. Color perception changes with age. The lens of the eye is yellow in all of us presumably to prevent chromatic aberration by inhibiting the passage of violet light. (Violet light bends more as it comes through the cornea and lens and is therefore relatively out of focus, blurring the retinal image.) The lens becomes more yellow with age. The world of an older person doesn't look yellow because the visual system adapts very quickly to overall coloration of illumination, but with less of the blue and violet light some facets of color vision and contour formation change. In addition, there is data showing that there are neural changes that lessen the effectiveness of violet light on the visual system.

It is possible to interact different kinds of wedges with one another. A yellow wedge can be positioned, together with a density wedge, on top of a letter-size wedge for example and combinations of these can be slid back and forth at right angles to simulate several factors and their interactions at once.

Many more of these practical physical, sensory, and motor simulations need to be developed. In cases of actual design these may work far better than psychophysical data from the laboratory or guidelines for design from the building codes. They can be performed on an individual basis and tested on the spot. Of course, after the sign is complete, the display is designed, the yellow marking on the stair is in place, be sure to verify that this end product is effective.

Mathematical models

In the past, mathematical models were primarily abstruse equations buried in books that were beyond normal comprehension. Now, because of the computer, they can be given interfaces and facilities for example for the collection of data that allow anyone to use them.

The type of mathematical model to be constructed and used is very dependent on the objectives for use of the model and the type of phenomenon to be studied. Are we doing a qualitative study or is some quantitative analysis of the problem at hand also possible?
Can we do some calculations?

Do we have to describe a phenomenon (which suggests using descriptive models), explain it (explanatory models) or do we want to make predictions about the future (predictive models/scenarios)? We must note that there does not necessarily exist a sharp distinction between these types of models.

Predictive models can be subdivided according to how cause and effect relationships are constructed in the model. These relationships inside the model do not necessarily correspond with those in the real world. Deterministic models state that cause A leads to effect B with complete security. For probabilistic models this is quite different: the response of the variables cannot be predicted with certainty.

Sometimes we find a fixed and time invariant probability that cause A leads to effect B, C, or D (implying probability models), sometimes probabilities vary over time but we know how time affects the probabilities (stochastic models) and sometimes we know that cause A has one of the effects B, C, or D but without knowing what the probability of occurrence of either one of these effects is (as in gambling or game theory models).

A special category of predictive models is comprised of the final-normative models that do not describe the reality of the present but the desired reality in the future. From this, one then can reason back to what should be done in the present.

Scenarios are an extension of models, being merely descriptions of possible developments in the future, mostly, but not always, based on model calculations. For scenarios it is essential that an eventual future situation is deducted from a well described starting situation that then might change in many different directions. Suggested changes can only be accepted in scenarios if they are consistent and plausible. Scenarios are specifically useful if they can be compared with other scenarios that are building upon the same starting situation. Scenarios can be divided into trend scenarios (trends from the past are used to predict the future) and normative scenarios (mostly used to solve political issues).

A warning about both the use of models and scenarios is called for here. In politics, science, and industrial organizations one often raises the question, "Which model or scenario is the basis of your statement?" This question should always be answered before thinking of building a model or a scenario for whatever challenging problem is to be attacked.

Mathematical models are not necessarily better than physical models (experimental and laboratory set-ups) or for that matter socio-economic models. They all have different strengths. Consider, for example, one of the main aspirations in gerontechnology, prediction.

Prediction with mathematical devices

The power of foresight is important in gerontechnology in many ways. "When will I need to have this joint replaced? What will happen and when will it happen if I continue on this diet, what form will my improvement take if I change diets? When will I be able to drive safely, and live independently again? What will the individual assistive devices add to my capability and safety in traffic?"

Ordinarily the trained intuition of a person, a physician or other practitioner, answers such questions. However, even though human intuition is very powerful in such matters, increasingly these are things that models and computers can do better than people can. However there is one massive prerequisite in the first step of building a model. The problem or situation at hand has to be assessed and identified (parametric model construction) properly.

Box 7.2 Four layer model

Several separate models can be "layered" together to form a comprehensive model. A four layer model of a human might be structured:

Layer 1. Physiological functioning of the body.

Layer 2. Physical performance, which could be estimated via performance of various exercises, physical skills, etc.

Layer 3. Cognitive performance of the individual that could be estimated by using some computerized tests or standard psychological tests.

Layer 4. Interactions with the world, situations, sequences, envelopes of performance and demand.

Thus, an integrated model of an individual here consists of four levels. This composite mathematical description encompassing all four levels allows us to diagnose, medically or otherwise, the state of the person in terms of the environment's influences, we can assess the need for medical or other treatment, we can regulate the microclimate in order to improve the person's circumstances (move the person's state from one location in the space of all possible states to some other, better, one).

A mathematical model in action can assimilate and process massive amounts of data, without forgetting any of it. A model can add endlessly to its own "training" by continuing to augment all of its databases. The models have the potential for "collective intellect" because they can be interconnected, sharing knowledge and experience over the existing communication networks faster and more extensively than people can.

And they can perform some inferential tasks, such as detecting the subtle effects of a number of interacting variables, better. As well, they can be made to operate more quickly in real-time in many cases. Humans are easily overloaded, and relatively easily confused when required to make complex correlations over time. It is difficult to recall what one had for breakfast two days ago, let alone recognize any effects of specific foods that are first emerging a day or two later. It is even less possible to realize that the effect only occurs when one has eaten extra salt, or perhaps eggs the previous day. The development of devices such as the Kalman filter, neural nets, and more modern models with their ability to take in immense amounts of data has astounding potential for older people.

The powerful mathematics of control systems

One of the most thriving areas of mathematical modeling is in the control of complex systems such as chemical plants, nuclear reactors, space ships, and even patients under anesthesia. These models are very good at handling systems with many dynamically changing variables and can be used to track changes in human physiological systems and suggest interjections that can stabilize and control them. We need much more effort in this direction in gerontechnology.

People are very dynamic. But as we age, our biological processes lose some of their original choreographing. They don't work in synchrony as well and so they must be artificially controlled. Mathematical models from control systems are perfect. They just need to be developed, tested, and applied.

Consider a few examples. Many of the diseases to which older people become more susceptible wax and wane unpredictably based on factors that are often difficult to discern and correlate. Diseases of the joints and the accompanying pain depend in complexly interacting ways on diverse factors such as specific foods in the diet, and the weather. The blood sugar of the diabetic presently must be tested very frequently because there are simply too many factors that influence it throughout the day.

Even though most of the vulnerabilities may be known, they haven't been adequately modeled. To illustrate, it has been shown in a massive public health study that diabetics should narrow their ranges of allowable blood sugar levels by employing closer monitoring and control–and this course of action is proscribed for older people because it is too dangerous for them to operate so close to the limits. Facts such as this virtually shout for control-oriented mathematical models to improve the prospects for regulation of bodily functioning.

Representative problems with typical modeling

Does the model fit?

No matter how exact a model may be, it still is a model and not completely identical to the entity that it is modeling. So, it may behave differently than its alter ego from time to time and probably will be somewhat discrepant all of the time. This is the issue of "fit." How closely does the behavior of the mathematical model parallel that of the system? Is it close enough for this application? Is it reliable, or does it wander off unpredictably from time to time? Only testing will tell you.

Lending your intuition to the model

A model must be initially "clued in" with some guesses about what the various variables that it will be watching will do in the future. For example, the "Kalman gains matrix" is a matrix of indices of confidence in the predictive reliability of each individual variable–how tightly related to blood sugar has heart rate been? When the variable, or one of its interactions with other variables, changes, how certain can we be that the state of the system will change accordingly? The model develops such numbers over time as it gains experience with the variables. So, in the beginning the model builder must assign some start-up values. They may be based on experimentation, they may be based on intuition, or they may be set arbitrarily. In each case, the hope is that the model will figure out better values as time passes and it accumulates experience.
Perhaps in a model that monitors ambulation, the predictive value of step length, moment-to-moment friction between the sole and the floor, and stubbing of the shoe interact so that stubbing the toe is only threatening and predictive of a fall if the friction is high and the length of step is short. Initially the model will not know this and will make mistakes about it until it figures out what is going on.

Box 7.3 Simulation of aging in the house

The dimensions of aging, as they bear on housing, are typically difficult to characterize in practice because every older person and every population of older people is different, as we have noted in many contexts. Older people may become weaker, perhaps very weak, or perhaps not very weak. They may lose endurance or not, have dizzy spells or not, or may have restricted ranges of motion of the joints—each profile of problems related to a house is different from all of the others.

Again we are led back to three possible solutions, first a mathematical model with which to characterize and customize the house so that its envelopes of tolerance enclose the envelopes of potential behaviors and sensitivities of possible older dwellers.

Second, some of the effects of sensory/motor decline can be assessed and corrected by employing the methods for simulating the dimensions of aging by putting restrictive devices directly on the person (Harrington et al., 1998.).

Third, the environment in the house can be altered to mimic the way that the older person has to perceive and deal with it. Requirements of torque and linear force can be elevated by stiffening up the motions of faucet handles, doorknobs, drawers, cupboard locks, medicine bottles and other items. Then "walk-throughs" of the house can be performed in which questions about the safety of the sequential situations an older person might encounter are asked. For instance, would expending so much energy on the "stiff" doorknob predispose one to momentarily losing cutaneous sensibility and strength of grip, leading to a misplaced and weakened grasp of the railing, and a fall down the stairs?

It must be kept in mind that even though the person experiencing the simulation may be climbing the stairs and dealing with the other aspects of the house with the same degree of inflexibility and impairment that the older person may have, the student still may have better balance, keener awareness, and better skills for recovering from a trip. Certainly they will also have more motivation to perform and to pay attention on this one time basis as subjects than residents may always have.

Harrington, T., Graafmans, J., Hermens, Y. & Weerd, W. de. (1998). Shade tree psychophysics: Models, mathematical and concrete, for the simulation of ageing. In: J.A.M. Graafmans, V. Taipale & N. Charness. (Eds.). Gerontechnology: A sustainable investment in the future. (pp. 115-117). IOS Press, Amsterdam. ISBN 90-5199-367-6.

Models require maturation to gain common sense

Hopefully, the models will eventually learn and get a handle on the situation; however, at times they don't. Especially during initial testing it is not uncommon for the model to "diverge," as the mathematicians put it, to wander farther and farther from the truth, until it "blows up," as the engineers say. This only means that the model decides that longevity is solely a matter of what kind of tooth paste you use or something similar. Blowing up isn't usually dangerous unless the model is involved in some critical monitoring and control procedure.

A model that blows up may recover or may just become unstable and stop functioning with any semblance of reality. A model may or may not have common sense with respect to its failings, so human common sense is sometimes needed, especially in the early stages of development.

Matching the parameters of older people

Most mathematical models have parameters incorporated in them. The word, parameter, means "parallel measure." In mathematical modeling it refers to a quantity, such as the height of a person, that is constant for the case under consideration, but that changes from case to case. In other words, a parameter is simply a characteristic.

So one must ask whether the parameters of the model are appropriate for older people. Is the model valid for older people? Existing models for a wide array of problems are valid for younger people, but not for seniors, so they need to be extended to fit them too. Standards for automobile safety and devices such as seat belts and airbags have been derived based on the "survival" of crash dummies. These have been constructed to model the human body–but, the body of a younger human–the parameters such as flexibility, breakability, and so on are wrong. Seniors are more frail and their crash dynamics are different. We have seen what air bags designed using models based on the parameters of adults do to children.

Similarly, the mouse, the guinea pig, the monkey, the rabbit, the baboon and many other animals have been used as "animal" models of human physiology to test the harmful, and the beneficial effects of drugs. Because older people are more susceptible to side effects and respond to pharmaceutical agents differently, these models too need to be reworked.

The language of mathematical modeling

Time scale

A mathematical model can operate on any time scale whatsoever. This opens up an amazing array of problems that we can deal with. We simply adjust the model to consider data on the time scale of the process that we are interested in, and set the model to talk to us in the range of time scales, very small, that humans can deal with.

Whereas events happen rather quickly in ambulation with a trip and fall occupying on the order of one second, we have to slow the model down so that we can see what's happening. On the other hand many of the changes from aging occur quite slowly so we have to speed the model up to view the panoramas of change. For instance, "accidents" such as Parkinsonism take much time to develop.

Changes in handwriting take place over a course of years, yet the dynamics of actual handwriting are much faster than those of walking. Making a mathematical model of a person's handwriting in terms of both the moment-to-moment movements as well as the slow changes of these motions and their coordination with age is quite feasible and may hold the key to developing some long-term diagnostic methods. In the case of Parkinson's disease for instance, people develop micrographia; they gradually begin to write smaller. Precursors of other tremors that are presently undetected in the handwriting signals may show up gradually too. The coordination of muscles and motions in handwriting are fairly critical and it would be expected that they provide advance windows on what the nervous system is going to do down the road.

The interface–how your model talks to you

Only a few years ago the language of mathematics was inappropriate for general use in complex problems such as those relating to older people. Tangled equations were limited to predicting and managing a few of the more tractable physical and economic processes. They were difficult to implement with only primitive computers, or without any at all, and impossible for the untrained to understand.

Presently however, because we have the technology to recast the language of models into the form of computer programs, we can construct "shells" around them. These are programs that can interface smoothly with untrained users. The shells can be very easy to understand and to interact with.

This gives the gerontechnologist a way to present this technological power to the practitioners and to older people themselves. It also creates another job for gerontechnologists: after a model is built, someone has to design the interface so that it is comprehensible to whoever will be using it.

Pie in the sky models

What are a few kinds of models that we might wish for? How about a model of optimal human functioning that watches us operate our computers, watches the times between key strokes, the pauses, the tremor of the mouse, mouse reaction times, the overshoots when we try to hit the buttons, and a thousand other things and tells us when we should or shouldn't try to be creative, write, drive, make important phone calls, try to learn new things?

A general model of mental functioning could monitor memory, cognitive skills, attention, and motor performance over the years too and sense changes and anticipate problems. Combining models of performance of the aged with models of tasks would allow not only prediction of which tasks a person could perform adequately. It would indicate precisely what a person would need to do in order to perform a given task that had become impossible, and indicate how more tractable sub-tasks could be incorporated to allow performance of the impossible tasks.

A comprehensive model of digestion is needed in gerontechnology. The model should deal with digestion at every internal stage in terms of each of the organs and systems that are related to metabolism. It should provide the power to predict the effects of diet hour-by-hour and year-by-year, and it should be sweepable. It should be possible to sweep it through the ages, youth through old age, and watch the changes on a display of organs and processes. It should be tunable to an individual's unique metabolic patterns, conditions and problems.

The steps in building a mathematical model

Usually, building a new complex special purpose model will require a mathematician. Often, during the first meetings, the gerontechnologist will not know what the mathematician has to offer or even what the problem actually is in terms of things that mathematics can grapple with. Similarly, the mathematician may not have a clear idea of what the goals are, where to start, what questions to ask, or what types of model may apply. Hopefully, some consideration of the specific steps that are usually necessary will help you through this phase. Warning: The steps required for building a good mathematical model can be laborious:

1. Structural identification. The mathematician identifies the optimal (or at least an adequate) structure (type of model), set of equations, etc., based on conversations with you, and perhaps based on preliminary data that is collected to assess roughly how the system under study can be expected to behave.

2. Data collection. Experimental measurements are made for estimating the coefficients of the model. What is the reaction time of the older person? How much force can they exert with one finger in turning a key?

3. Validity testing. The mathematician matches the model's behavior to the data that has been collected. Usually it is required that the model be able to perform at or above some criterion level, perhaps a minimum mean square error. [The mean square error is a summation of all the squared errors (these are discrepancies between what the model predicts and what actually happens, squared so that they won't cancel each other when they are summed), divided by the number of them to arrive at their mean.]

4. Refinement. This phase needs to be carried out if the model isn't sufficiently valid. The experimental data may have been collected incorrectly, the experimental design for collecting data may have been inappropriate, the model may not in fact be the right one for this application, or the numerical procedure for coefficient (parameters of the model) estimation may contain errors. This step to some extent is a mathematics/engineering art based on experience, knowledge, and intuition.

Some of the language of modeling

Classes of dynamic system models

The landscape of possible models for use in gerontechnology is growing every day, so choosing the best model for some application, in collaboration with one's mathematician offers many options. In Table 7.1 some of the choices are shown. These choices need to be made in order to fit the experimental problem with a model.

Table 7.1 General characteristics of dynamic system models

Time discrete. (Blood sugar, thyroid level.) Occasional measurement.	Time-continuous. (Ambulation blood sugar.) Continuous measurement.
Time variant. (Aging itself.) Our parameters change.	Time invariant. (Short-term problems.) Where the parameters don't change–bone density.
Linear dynamics. (Another day another dollar.)	Non-linear dynamics. (Human temperament.)
Single-input Single-output (SISO). (A target to be tracked vs. position of the eye or hand.)	Multi-input Multi-output. (MIMO.) (Aspects of mood depending on many factors; microclimate in a house.)
Lumped parameters. (blood pressure.) Different everywhere but lumped into one average value.	Distributed parameters. (Skin temperature.) Measured all over the skin.
Parametric. (Strength.) Parameters are explicit in the model.	Non-parametric. (Blood pressure/salt intake.) No parameters in the model, e.g. just a correlation between things.
Deterministic. (Relation of pulse to exercise with no random variation considered.) Has no random variables.	Stochastic. (Equation for arrival time of the bus.) Has random variables that take on different variables unpredictable but with known probability.
Single layer. (Person's physiology alone.)	Hierarchical. (Person's cognitive state as underlied by their physiology.)
Causal. (Stroke as caused by blood pressure and weakened arteries.) Definite causes and effects.	Non-causal. (Model of style of walking, slumped etc.) No causes and effects.
One-dimensional. (Velocity of ambulation.) Single dimension of description.	Two or more dimensional. (Velocity of walking and step frequency.)
Non-fuzzy. (Monthly income.) Only regular numerical variables.	Fuzzy. (Feelings–I feel fair.) Contains linguistic variables.
Simplified. (Dynamics of brain's storage.) Doesn't reflect the nature of the actual process–just a differential equation or some such.	Imitational. (Brain's storage of information/computer.) Part of the model, e.g. computer memory, mimics the brain's storage.

Suggested readings

Harrington, T., Graafmans, J., Hermens, Y. & Weerd, W. de. (1998). Shade tree psychophysics: Models, mathematical and concrete, for the simulation of ageing. In: J.A.M. Graafmans, V. Taipale & N. Charness. (Eds.). Gerontechnology: A sustainable investment in the future. (pp. 115-117). IOS Press, Amsterdam. ISBN 90-5199-367-6.

Schieber, F. (1992). Aging and the senses. In: J.E. Birren, R.B. Sloane & G.D. Cohen (Eds.). Handbook of mental health and aging. Academic Press, San Diego. ISBN 0-12-101277-8.

Tsang, P.F. & Shaner, T.L. (1998). Age, attention, expertise and time-sharing performance. Psychology and Aging, 13, 323-347.

Suggested websites

http://www.cis.upenn.edu/~hms/home.html
Center for Human Modeling and Simulation of the University of Pennsylvania.

http://www.lasiksafety.com/VisionPlaceIII/discover/vissim.htm
Website with a Vision Simulator, showing you how a variety of different conditions could change your vision.

CHAPTER EIGHT
Gerontechnology unfolding

Let's start the concluding chapter with a question. Do you wish to become very old? Supposedly it depends. If you stay reasonably healthy then you won't mind. If you still have family and friends then it's no problem. Moreover, if you can continue to live independently then you won't mind either. And if your health should fail, then you want to have good care. In brief, you wish to live a long life, but you want favorable conditions for it.

Among such conditions is a favorable technological environment. In the rich countries, much of the technology has become so obvious that we don't even consider it any more. For a hundred years we have had electric lighting, for 70 years we have had radios, and for 50-60 years we have had television sets and telephones, and more recently mobile phones. We have central heating, there is a microwave oven in the kitchen, and there is a car outside the door. When we become old we want to hold onto this technology even if we aren't that technical ourselves.

Some maintain that older people are afraid of technology. After having read this book, you will not agree. Older citizens use technology every day, just like everybody else. Technology provides comfort and gives people means for mobility, communication, and recreation. We like life's little luxuries and these luxuries generally rely on technology. So there's no fear of technology as such; perhaps there is only a certain amount of suspicion about the usefulness of specific innovations, a personal weighing of costs and benefits, and some awkwardness with it at the beginning.

Let's take a closer look at this awkwardness. Awkwardness is connected to the newness of things that are not part of the daily routine. To put it scientifically, there is a discrepancy between which useful products are available in society and which have actually been realized for certain groups. The discrepancy usually leaves older people trailing. And the faster society changes, the greater the discrepancy becomes.

The threat is that older citizens can no longer participate as full citizens in their own society (Lawton, 1998).

Age as a culture-determining factor is a recent phenomenon. Demographic developments favoring the old, and technological environments favoring the young, have drifted apart. Effective coping with the daily environment is at the core of social theories on aging.

Electronic mail (e-mail) provides an example. In science and industry, e-mail has recently become as indispensable as the telephone. E-mail is easy and interactive. Larger documents are distributed via e-mail too, although most people start to read them only after printing. Unfortunately, not all older people presently use e-mail. The older people that do are enthusiastic about it. E-mail is an example of a useful service, which will probably take some years to come into general use by older people. There are several reasons for this: unfamiliarity with the function, high price, and difficult access. One thing that might work toward increasing the success would be refraining from referring to it as a computer service.
The word computer may act to some as an additional barrier.

But we need a better analysis. E-mail conquered the professional world in the early nineties. Most older people are not familiar with e-mail from their professional lives. They do not know the advantages from personal experience. Furthermore, you have to be able to type to use e-mail presently, and that's not something everybody learned in the past. So most older people will have to learn this later in life. And finally, e-mail is still tied to a PC, which is expensive and difficult to buy in some countries, not sturdily built, and hard to use. On the positive side, the e-mail addresses are easier to remember than telephone numbers or postal codes, but you only notice this when you actually start using e-mail.

The example of e-mail is relatively simple. A more complex example is the information network that we refer to as the World Wide Web or simply the web. The user threshold for the Internet is higher than for e-mail because the search process can be rather complicated. The information you require may be hidden in a lot of non-information or, worse, in deliberately distracting advertisements. In searching, you may have to look at things you are not interested in. In addition, waiting times can be so lengthy that you give up.

Box 8.1 Technology generations

In sociology, a concept of generation has been developed that is different from calendar age. The older people of today are not similar to the old of 10 to 20 years ago and the older citizens in the coming 10 to 20 years will be different again. This is because of their different life experiences (Glenn, 1977).

Generations are formed as a result of discontinuous changes in the social environment such as those resulting from wars, economic depressions, migrations, and similar radical changes in society that people born in certain years (birth cohorts) have to live through. Particularly the life period between 10 and 25 years seems to be a sensitive one; these years are taken as the formative period since the experiences during that period of becoming an independent person appear to have a lasting effect. We therefore refer to the pre-war generation, the baby boom generation, etc. The present generation of older people often had quite a number of children though many of them now live further away from their parents' homes. Education has gradually risen in the past century. This has resulted in changes in the types of jobs held and the work experiences of older people, both for men and women.

In a similar vein, we are presently considering technology generations: the experiences we gain by dealing with certain technologies when we are young are shaping our attitudes toward similar or dissimilar technologies that appear later in life (van de Goor & Becker, 2000). Referring to consumer appliances in Europe, we may speak of the mechanical generation (born before 1930), the electro-mechanical generation (born between 1930 and 1960) and the digital generation (born after 1960) (Docampa Rama & van der Kaaden, in press).

Docampo Rama, M. & Kaaden, F. van der. (in press). Technology generations: characterisation on the basis of user interface changes. Proceedings of the 3rd International Congress on Gerontechnology, Munich.

Glenn, N.D. (1977). Cohort analysis. Sage Publications, Beverley Hills. ISBN 0-8039-0794-X.

Goor, A.G. van de & Becker, H.A. (2000). Technology generations in the Netherlands: a social analysis. Shaker, Maastricht.

If we want to make e-mail or the web or other useful functions of ICT available on a wide scale for older citizens, then we have a number of tasks.

The first is focusing on functionalities rather than on PC's. We can isolate e-mail, the web or part thereof, and other useful functions from the overpowering functionality of the PC and offer it cheaply and separately. Removing such useful functions from their computer environment primarily is a task of industry. Work is being done at the moment. However, business and industry have been slow in providing useful products for the market of older people, possibly because they have elevated economic boundary conditions to be the main objective, rather than fulfilling their primary and essential task in society of providing suitable products and services.

This concluding chapter blends back into Chapter 1 in that the basics of gerontechnology are laid down once more. But here we emphasize the relationships with some of the neighboring multidisciplinary areas from which progress in technology for older people can be expected and from which relevant methods can be learned. These are concerned in particular with information ergonomics, assistive technology, and situated embedded learning systems. Since the main emphasis of gerontechnology is on ambitions and desires of older people themselves, we conclude with a section on technological opportunities for promoting good health, this being one of the most valued assets of older people.

Information ergonomics

We can increase the ease of use by developing a good user interface for older people. This primarily requires scientific research because we do not possess the knowledge to do this properly. The alterations necessary for older users include adaptations to sight, sound, memory, learning, attention, and motor skills. We do have the methodology. We can study the literature to know how perceptive, cognitive, and motor functions develop with age. We need to know more about the processes of learning, memorizing, and forgetting, as this occurs in older people.

> ## Box 8.2 Networking with other scientific organizations
>
> During the past years, gerontechnology has been on the agenda of many related scientific associations. This has been materialized in symposia, seminars, workshops, or key-notes on gerontechnology at a number of international conferences, such as:
> - International Ergonomics Association (IEA)
> - European Society for Engineering and Medicine (ESEM)
> - International Federation for Medical and Biological Engineering (IFMBE)
> - Institute of Electrical and Electronics Engineers (IEEE)
> - International Association of Gerontology (IAG)
> - Human Factors and Ergonomics Society (HFES)
> - Computer Human Interaction (CHI)
> - International Association for Person-environment Studies (IAPS)
> - Human Service Information Technology Applications (HUSITA)
> - European Gerontology Conference (EGC)
>
> In this way, opportunities were created to present gerontechnology projects within existing networks.

Let's take the sharpness of eyesight, which grows weaker as we age, as an example. Low vision will be rather troublesome because a visual computer display consists of miniature pictograms, including text characters. A higher contrast between the letters and the background helps. If this isn't enough, we can increase the size of letters and icons though we know from the literature that large letters tend to slow down the reading process (Bouma, Legein, Mélotte & Zabel, 1982; Aberson & Bouwhuis, 1997). Another disadvantage of large letters is that less text fits onto the screen, which diminishes the global picture. So we need better solutions for the division of the screen. If large letters and higher contrast prove inadequate, we can have the text read out to us via speech synthesis; speech however is volatile while text on a screen remains visible. The choice of which text to say at which time, is another problem that has to be solved.

As to cognitive functions, disregarding specific diseases affecting memory, older people are capable of learning up to an advanced age, especially if the new knowledge is rooted in existing knowledge and skills. On the other hand, we know that the working memory deteriorates, as does the signaling function of the prospective memory (Craik & Bosman, 1992).

Information technology can compensate for this with a proper interaction protocol. So, on the basis of a task analysis that includes the user, an interface can be designed that makes optimal use of the stable human functions that don't change as the user ages and that compensates for functions that deteriorate with age (Bouma, 2000). It would be an adaptive interface that adjusts its settings semi-automatically to the needs of the user. For this to work, we will need to evaluate simulations and prototypes with carefully selected test persons from the target group.

The adaptation of such technical products and services to the user is an existing field called information ergonomics. What gerontechnology adds is the adaptation to the functions of the older user. Toward this purpose the concept of adaptive technology was developed in recent years, in which adaptations to the user or various kinds of user operate automatically or semi-automatically. Information ergonomics for older people is an extensive field of gerontechnology.

Assistive technology

For persons with functional impairments, particularly in mobility and motor functions, assistive technology has a long tradition in helping to minimize the resulting disabilities or even handicaps that threaten independence in daily life. In other areas such as vision and hearing, there have been similar developments. For people with low vision, for example, closed circuit television circuits for enlarging text and photographs have been developed, and for people that are hard of hearing, hearing aids have proven useful. For quite a few deficiencies, the likelihood of suffering from them increases with age. Other deficiencies, such as most color weaknesses or reading weakness (dyslexia) bear no specific relation to old age but rather to genetic factors. Assistive technology aims at improving the quality of life of all citizens that have to live with certain impairments (Placencia Porrero & Ballabio, 1998).

In as far as people with functional deficits are old, assistive technology for them can be taken as part of gerontechnology. However, the point of view of gerontechnology is a different one. Gerontechnology would rather emphasize the specific requirements that older people with certain impairments might have. These could be concerned with specific tasks or desires that would fit their ambitions, with specific situations such as a combination of sensory and motor difficulties, and with specific physical and social environments. For example, the recent digital hearing aids are more versatile, can better suppress noise, and operate largely automatically, thus relieving the users of the task of handling miniature control wheels such as for sound volume.

The gerontechnology approach has been amply dealt with in the preceding chapters, to which the reader is referred.

Situated, embedded learning

In order to acquaint people with ICT functions such as in using e-mail or searching the web, courses can be organized, including limited typing courses. This task is not primarily technical. Successful courses exist in many countries. However, they are more complex than necessary because of the dependence on the PC.

However, the learning process can be supported by technology. One of the conditions for efficient learning is to concentrate on things you need to learn as a learner and not to waste time on stuff you already know or things that are still too difficult or not yet necessary. These conditions can be built into flexible technological systems as powerful tools for older people, helping them to gain skills and knowledge in many fields. So, courses for e-mail and for the web can be simplified by building into the equipment training programs specifically targeted at older people. These are available as one goes, efficient, and easy to fall back on if you haven't worked with the equipment for a while. You always have additional training at hand. Learning as you go is also referred to as situated learning. Thus we are able to provide powerful technological support to the user where and when it is really needed (Masthoff, 1997).

The development of situated learning program with a generic user interface for the continuous development of older people is another exciting field of gerontechnology.

Box 8.3 Some programs in Europe

European Union (EU).

Program "Ageing and Technology" (COST A5 1991-1996)

This started after the 1st conference on gerontechnology in Eindhoven under the auspices of European Cooperation in Science and Technology in which 25 European countries participate. The leading idea of COST A5 was that the needs, preferences, and potentialities of the growing population of older people needed greater attention.

COST A5 has explored conditions for extended autonomy, independence, and activity for older people in a European comparative perspective. It led to conferences on mobility, housing, health, design, and gerontechnology education, all with useful reports, and formed the basis for the International Society for Gerontechnology (ISG).
The network was instrumental in the JRC-study, "The state of the art in ageing and technology" and the ETAN-expert group on "Ageing and Technology." COST A5 has been instrumental in getting "Ageing and Technology" on the agenda of the 5th Framework Program.

Design for Ageing Network (DAN)

DAN is mainly concerned with developing the necessary expertise, know-how, and understanding to enable design and industry to respond to the growing population of over-50's in Europe in life-enhancing ways. One important element in DAN's approach to design is its in-depth collaboration with older people. For example, in the UK DAN works together with the dynamic University of the 3rd Age (U3A), run by and for older people.

Eurolink Age Subgroup on Ageing and Technology

This subgroup was established in 1998 and aims at reviewing and advising on specific aspects of policy relating to older people across Europe. The focus is on education and training, issues of older workers, social protection and care, technology and housing for the domain of gerontechnology.

GENIE (1998-2001)

Forty institutes from sixteen countries participate in GENIE: Gerontechnology Education Network In Europe. GENIE is a 3-year project. After the 3rd operational year it is envisaged to continue as a Standing Committee and Working Group within ISG.

The objective is to improve the quality of gerontechnology education, to increase the European dimension and to stimulate the acceptance of gerontechnology as a part of regular university programs. It will encourage the interaction between teaching staff and students and stimulate the dissemination of knowledge and the use of developed course materials.

The 5th Framework RTD Program of EU

Program "Quality of life and Management of living resources," key action "The Ageing Population"

The overriding goal of this key action is to promote quality of life and healthy ageing and independence in old age by preventing and treating age-related diseases and disability, and their societal consequences.
A complementary objective will be to reduce the need for long-term care and limit the constantly increasing costs of health-care systems.

Program "User friendly information society," key action "Systems and Services for the Citizen"

Health. Work will cover new generation computerized clinical systems, advanced telemedicine services and health network applications to support health professionals, continuity of care and health service management, and intelligent systems allowing citizens to assume greater participation and responsibility for their own health.

Persons with special needs, such as older people. Work will address person/system interfaces and adaptive and assistive systems to overcome problems caused by environmental barriers and by physical or intellectual impairments, as well as intelligent systems and services to support autonomous living, social integration, and participation in the information society.

Saranummi, N. (1997). Ageing and technology. State of the Art.
European Commission Joint Research Centre, Sevilla. EUR 17285 EN.

EU 5th framework program. http://www.cordis.lu/fp5/src/programmes.htm

DAN. http://dan.interact.nl

Technology supporting ambitions of older people

We started out our final exploration with the new services presented in society, which take a long time to penetrate the world of older people. We now take an entirely different perspective, the aspirations and wishes of the older citizens themselves. If we map both the aspects of life that older people value and the products and services that would help, we can go on to consider which new technological means there are and which investments and savings are concerned.

Such mapping is not an easy task because it requires the imagination to sketch older people of a certain generation in an environment that is not yet here and that comes from the technical world that, to many, is not familiar. The general theoretical basis has been laid down earlier. Lewin (1951) discussed the important role of the environments or fields in which actions of people take place. Lawton (1989) discussed the interaction between person and environment in terms of potentialities and restrictions of the person, and opportunities and constraints of the environment.
Baltes & Baltes (1990) concentrated on what persons do when they have to tone down their aspirations, choosing between full compensation, assimilation, and accommodation. The latter implies that the new condition is accepted as unavoidable (Brandstädter & Renner, 1990). However, it is only recently that the technical environment for such decisions has been addressed as such (Lawton, 1998; Slangen-de Kort, 1999).

So, there is a problem here. Technology is developing so rapidly that it is practically impossible for older people to say exactly which innovations they would appreciate. There is a gap between the young professionals on the forefront of hardware and software technology and interface design on the one hand, and the many potential older users of this technology on the other. To bridge this gap, gerontechnology employs its methodological approach, integrating the relevant methodologies of the technical, biological, and social research disciplines.

We include the following fields as relevant life domains for older people: health; one's home (and its safety and security); mobility outdoors (private and public transportation); information and communication; professional work, voluntary work, and hobbies; and recreation and relaxation. You will find this list closely reflected in the preceding chapters. Priorities within these lists as experienced by older people are globally known, but differ between persons, groups, and cultures. That is why target groups must be involved and that is why we need them to evaluate simulations, prototypes, and experimental systems, because the products and services have to be suitable for living environments and living patterns of older people. Examples from the field of mobility (see Chapter 5) include an experimental system of city buses that is not aimed at speed but at comfort and that has a high density of bus stops, and a city transport system that can be accessed at home, allowing you to find out when the next bus is coming to the nearest bus stop.

Health technology or Public Health Engineering

We will work out the example of the health domain (see also Chapter 2), because we know older people attach high priority to proper health. There is an interesting historical parallel. In the 20th century in industrial countries the average life expectancy at birth has almost doubled. The spectacular gain is mainly due to technology: improved hygiene through safe water systems and closed sewers, improved ways of preparing and storing food, improved labor conditions, and so on. We call this health technology or Public Health Engineering.

To make things more concrete for the present situation of older people, we can turn to future expectations for public health. In the Netherlands, for example, these are being published every five years, lastly in 1997.
We find lists of the most prevalent diseases among older people, which are often of a chronic nature. We see that the margins of health decrease for older people as they continue to age, and the probability grows of having more diseases simultaneously. The diseases described have various natures, including sensory limitations such as failing eyesight and deafness. From an economic perspective we find the costs of health care connected to the occurrence and prevention of these diseases and of their consequences.

Living environment and behaviour can influence a number of these diseases. Examples are osteoporosis in relation to nutrition, allergic diseases in relation to the indoor and outdoor climate, and limitations in mobility in relation to daily activity.

Box 8.4 International Society for Gerontechnology (ISG)

ISG was established in 1997 as a non-profit organization for promoting gerontechnology as a forum for discussion and action and for promoting interdisciplinary projects within all countries and across boundaries. Following the 1st international conference in Eindhoven (1991) and the 2nd in Helsinki (1996), ISG has taken responsibility for a regular series of international gerontechnology conferences: Munich (1999), Miami (2002), and probably Japan (2005).

Objectives of ISG include:

- Promoting cultural and scientific international exchanges among engineers, researchers, designers, architects, and professionals in industry and in the fields of comfort, welfare, and health for the aging and the aged;
- Encouraging the creation of international research networks;
- Promoting international experiments of an applied nature, in order to reinforce international potentialities in gerontechnology and to participate in their assessment;
- Promoting international programs in gerontechnology;
- Reinforcing the participation of engineers, vocational professionals, administrators and industrial management in specific educational training courses in the domain of gerontechnology;
- Co-operating closely with all similar international organizations and with all national bodies, governmental and non-governmental, concerned with gerontechnology;
- Involving older citizens and their organizations in all relevant activities.

To reach these objectives, the following seven standing committees have been established: Publication; Internal and External Communication; Education; Research, Design and Development; Industrial relations; and Conferences. The committees formulate and implement working plans thus supporting the tasks of the Council. The primary objective of the Council itself will be the further development and promotion of gerontechnology.

http://www.gerontechnology.org
Website of the International Society for Gerontechnology.

Let's take a closer look at activity. The optimal daily activity is not the same for everybody and depends on a number of physiological factors, like body weight and condition of the muscles, the cardio-vascular system, and the lungs. Too little activity is a danger to muscles and joints, too much activity endangers heart and lungs. We could measure the daily activity via a system with a small 3-D acceleration sensor, and compare the obtained values to an individual target value. As a result we can give feedback to the user telling him to be more active or less active. In this way we can also realize gradual training for improved fitness. Research has shown this possible up to a very high age. In addition, warnings can be issued in the event of high stress, as may occur during jogging when people want to perform too well.

For professional athletes most ingredients for such a performance monitor are available. But the application as a health monitor for older people does not exist: the reliable recording of individual target values, entering this into equipment, comfort of use, suitable forms of feedback and warnings, introduction into health care, and the evaluation of all this by the target group, we are still waiting for.

In a similar fashion monitors can be designed for other aspects of health. How about a simple sensor to detect the beginnings of food decay for products in the fridge such as a sticker that discolors? Or why not have a medicine cabinet that keeps track of the use of medicine and the proper dosages, that warns you if something is going wrong or reminds you to use vitamins or food supplements? Of course the co-operation of the user is a prerequisite.

Health education: timely and tailored

Health information could really use a push. At present it lacks focus. It lies around in waiting rooms or reaches us through advertisements on television. Though everybody may have been warned, it comes as no surprise that it is not effective. We can work far more precisely nowadays. To this purpose we need to map two kinds of risk factors.

Box 8.5 Gerontechnology research across the world

Answering the demands of an aging population several research projects or research centers were established all around the world. The examples described in this box illustrate such initiatives.

CREATE: Center for Research and Education on Aging and Technology Enhancement

Participants in this project, funded by the National Institute on Aging (1999-2003), include the University of Miami, Florida State University, and Georgia Institute of Technology, USA. The goal is to enhance computer interaction for older adults through three projects.

The first project focuses on understanding how to facilitate performance in tasks that involve information search and retrieval such as searching the WWW, and querying databases.

In the second project, the emphasis is on understanding input devices, particularly how to facilitate interaction via mouse, light pen, speech recognition, and in tasks that require voice input and output.

Third, uncovering principles for effective training for computer applications (e.g., web browsers) by understanding how age-related changes in cognitive factors influence learning to use technology will be studied.

MIT's AgeLab: Ideas and Technology for Healthy Aging

This research lab at MIT promotes healthy independent living throughout the human lifespan. Based in the School of Engineering, the AgeLab is a partnership between MIT, industry and the aging community to pioneer new technologies, which respond to the needs and preferences of older adults, their families, and their care providers. The research program is based on a number of scientific disciplines, including engineering, computer science, planning and management, as well as the health and social sciences. The general objective is to reengineer the physical environment to enable people to enjoy an active life as long as possible.

One of the focus areas will be lifelong transportation–the use of technology to provide a continuum of attractive transportation alternatives as we age. Other areas of inquiry include "healthy home" research to explore the uses of technology for safety and well-being throughout the spectrum of housing alternatives; personal communications; research to define the older adult and caregiver markets for advanced interactive personal communications systems and productive workplace research to address the needs of older workers.

HQL: Institute of Human Engineering for Quality Life. Osaka, Japan.
The Research Institute of Human Engineering for Quality Life was established to undertake research and development, conduct surveys, and compile and disseminate information related to human life engineering.
The current research activities focus on Behavior-Based Human Technology (1999-2003). The project aims to develop systems that are compatible with natural human behavior for creating safe and comfortable environments. It uses new approaches to human-oriented technology and analysis of a variety of human functions. Three major research themes are:
Technologies for measuring human behavior;
Technologies for understanding and accumulation of measured behavior, and assisting human behavior;
Technologies for creating behavior based human environments.

GGT: Gesellschaft für Gerontotechnik, Iserlohn, Germany
The "Gesellschaft für Gerontotechnik" provides the integrative power necessary to stimulate cooperation between Industry, Science, and Consumers. In 1997 the Center for Gerontechnology was established, a business center aiming at the further development of gerontechnology through bringing together new, innovative companies. The Center provides a platform for discussion between the developers of technology, the older consumers, and the scientists. Part of the Center is an exhibition where examples of products that facilitate active aging are demonstrated. A panel of over 600 older people is available and frequently asked to give their opinion about new products, to do user tests, or to fill in questionnaires.

http://www.psy.fsu.edu/~charness/create/
Website of the CREATE project.

http://web.mit.edu/agelab/index.html
Website of MIT's AgeLab, Ideas and Technology for Healthy Aging.

http://www.hql.or.jp/gpd/eng/www/index.html
Website of the Research Institute of Human Engineering for Quality of Life.

http://www.gerontotechnik.de/
Website of the Gesellschaft für Gerontotechnik.

The first kind is in the living environment. One example is concerned with the qualities of the outdoor environment and the indoor environment. We refer to qualities in the plural, because there are several factors that can be detrimental, such as nitrogen oxides, carbon monoxide or tobacco smoke, and also biological factors like bacteria, fungi, and mites. We really need to introduce as a public standard requirement a health effect report on the living environment with an epidemiological focus, next to an environmental effect report.

A second kind of risk factor is the individual difference in sensitivity or vulnerability, because of predisposition, former exposure in the working environment, or through living habits. Examples are heightened sensitivity to mite excrements or to certain pets for asthma sufferers, or deafness through former exposure to loud noise. Age often is an important parameter.

If we provide information at the moment the combination of living environment and personal disposition becomes unhealthy, we gain prevention just in time, just in place, and tailored to the individual. We need new technological systems that can warn us, and if desired can advise us how to change our environments and our behaviors to regain a healthy situation.

The more we know which people are predisposed to have certain illnesses or ailments and which environmental factors play a role, the more we can develop helpful monitoring systems that scan the environmental factors for people. And nowadays we know more about which people run higher risks because of their genetic constitution, existing illnesses, age, etc. Moreover, we also know which environmental factors can have a positive or negative impact.

Adding this to the means of communication with experts in the field of health, e.g. through e-mail, this may mean a considerable shift from curative to preventive medicine. As older people have a higher risk of health problems, developments in this field would be most welcome. The tailored health information also belongs to the new field within gerontechnology, which is referred to as public health engineering.

Summarizing

Generalizing from the example of health, we can make an analysis for each of the other important life aspects of older people, e.g. safety, security, communication, mobility, travel, housing, work, relaxation, hobbies. For all of these, we have to take into account the desires and ambitions of older people as well as their living environments, their constitutions, and their habits. We will then be able to find out which technology is suitable for developing the right products and services.

To increase their control over the environment, they need properly designed and easy interfaces. We should avoid adding another five remote controls. We want a universal and generic user interface with powerful feedback and effective means to provide choices. These have to operate in the same way for all applications and be able to automatically adapt to the user in the environment through in-built agents.

Such an approach based on the ambitions and living environments of older people provides access to several fields of innovative gerontechnology research. The result is an improved quality of life for older people and support for independent living.

Both society as a whole and older citizens themselves have to get used to the realities of life-long learning. Life-long learning does not stop at 27 or 45, but indeed lasts a lifetime. All citizens should be encouraged and given the opportunity to keep up with the dynamics of the information society.

Older people have taught us that technology has to be situated, focused on the target group, and made suitable for individual and social environments. Institutes that allocate funds for scientific research should take an integrated look at problems in society and not just focus on segmented disciplines. And those interested in controlling the costs of aging society and wanting to promote the quality of life, will have to invest in preventive technology with high social benefits. Socially, older people do not simply represent costs; they are a rich source of life experience and participation, which they often give to society for free. They are more than worthy of a social investment in the form of education and of research, development, and design. Organizations of older people will welcome such a gerontechnology approach and will use their influence for having it realized.

Finally, demographic and technological changes are not at all restricted to industrial countries, on which this book has largely focused. We feel that the efforts of gerontechnology should also be directed toward countries in a different phase of development. We very much hope that in the near future we will be able to report much progress in technology for an adequate quality of life for all older people of our planet.

Suggested readings

Anan, K.A. (2000). We the people. The role of the United Nations 21st century. United Nations, New York. ISBN 92-1-100844-1.

Campbell, P., Dries, J. & Gilligan, R. (1999). The older generation and the European information society: access to the information society. Final project report: Recommendations for policy makers, NGO's and industry. European Institute for the Media, Düsseldorf. ISBN 90-76299-04-8.

Charness, N. (Ed.). (1985). Aging and human performance: Studies in human performance. Wiley, New York. ISBN 0-471-90068-0.

Craik, F.I.M. & Salthouse, T.A. (2000). The Handbook of aging and cognition, 2nd Edition. Lawrence Erlbaum Associates, Publishers, Hillsdale, N.J. ISBN 0-8058-2966-0.

Czaja, S. & Glascock, A. (Eds.). (1994). Technology and environmental issues for the elderly. Experimental Aging Research, 20(3, Special issue). Taylor and Francis, Washington D.C. ISSN 0361-073X.

Fisk, A.D. & Rogers, W.A. (Eds.). (1996). Handbook of human factors and the older adult. Academic Press, San Diego. ISBN 0-12-257680-2.

Fozard, J.L., Rietsema, J., Bouma, H. & Graafmans, J.A.M. (2000, in press). Gerontechnology: Creating enabling environments for the challenge and opportunities of aging. Educational Gerontology.

Karwowski, W. (Ed.). (2000). International encyclopedia of ergonomics and human factors. Taylor and Francis, London. ISBN 0-7484-0847-9.

Rogers, W.A., Fisk, A.D. & Walker, N. (Eds.). (1996). Aging and skilled performance. Lawrence Erlbaum Associates, Publishers, Mahwah, N.J. ISBN 0-8058-1909-6.

Rowe, J.W. & Kahn, R.L. (1998). Successful aging. Pantheon Books, New York. ISBN 0-375-40045-1.

Saranummi, N. (1997). Ageing and technology: state of the art. European Commission Joint Research Centre, Sevilla. EUR 17285 EN.

World Health Organization. (1998). The World Health Report. Life in the 21st century: a vision for all. World Health Organization, Geneva. ISBN 92-4-156189-0.

Suggested websites

http://www.seniorweb.com
Website for senior citizens.

http://www.elderweb.org
On-line community of older adult computer users.

http://www.gerontechnology.org/
Website of the International Society for Gerontechnology.

Bibliography

AARP. (1992). Older driver skill assessment and resource guide. Creating mobility choices. American Association for Retired Persons, Washington, D.C.

Aberson, D.H. & Bouwhuis, D.G. (1997). Silent reading as determined by age and visual acuity. Journal of Research in Reading, 20, 184-204.

Anan, K.A. (2000). We the people. The role of the United Nations in the 21st century. United Nations, New York. ISBN 92-1-100844-1.

Ausman, L.M. & Russell, R.M. (1990). Nutrition and aging. In: E.L. Schneider & J. Rowe. (Eds.). Handbook of the biology of aging. 3rd Edition. (pp. 385-406). Academic Press, New York. ISBN 0-87893-043-4.

Bailer, J.C. & Mosteller, F. (Eds.). (1986). Medical uses of statistics. New England Journal of Medicine Books, Waltham, MA. ISBN 0-910133-16-6.

Ball, K., Owsley, C., Thomas, B. & Graves, M. (1995). Predictors of useful field of view test performance. The Gerontologist, 35 (Special Issue 1), 365.

Baltes, P.B. & Baltes, M.M. (1990). Successful aging: Perspectives from the behavioural sciences. Cambridge University Press, Cambridge. ISBN 0-521-37454-5.

Bezooijen, C.F.A. van. (1996). Biological ageing, theories of ageing, age-associated diseases and their intervention. In: W.J.A. Goedhard. (Ed.). Aging and Work 3. (pp.19-34). ICOH Scientific Committee Aging and Work, [S.l.]. ISBN 90-803145-1-X.

Birren, J.E. (Ed.). (1996). Encyclopedia of gerontology: Age, aging and the aged. Academic Press, London. ISBN 0-12-226860-1.

Birren, J.E. & Schaie, K.W. (Eds.). (1995). Handbook of the psychology of aging. 4th Edition. Academic Press, San Diego. ISBN 0-122-101261-1.

Blaich, R.I. (1992). Taming technology for the benefit of the aging - and everyone else. In: H. Bouma & J.A.M. Graafmans. (Eds.). Gerontechnology. (pp. 7-14). IOS Press, Amsterdam. ISBN 90-5199-072-3.

Bouma, H., Legein, Ch.P., Mélotte, H.E.M. & Zabel, L. (1982). Is large print easy to read? IPO Annual Progress Report, 17, 84-90.

Bouma, H. (1992). Gerontechnology: Making technology relevant for the elderly.
In: H. Bouma & J.A.M. Graafmans. (Eds.). Gerontechnology. (pp. 1-5).
IOS Press, Amsterdam. ISBN 90-5199-072-3.

Bouma, H. & Graafmans, J. (Eds.). (1992). Gerontechnology. Proceedings of the first
International Conference on Gerontechnology, Eindhoven, August 1991.
IOS Press, Amsterdam. ISBN 90-5199-072-3.

Bouma, H. (1998). Gerontechnology: Emerging technologies and their impact on aging
in society. In: J. Graafmans, V. Taipale & N. Charness. (Eds.).
Gerontechnology: A sustainable investment in the future. (pp. 93-104).
IOS Press, Amsterdam. ISBN 90-5199-367-6.

Bouma, H. (2000). Document and user interface design for older citizens.
In: P.H. Westendorp, C.J.M. Jansen & R. Punselie. (Eds.). Interface design and
document design. Rodopi Press, Amsterdam. ISBN 90-420-0510-6.

Bouwhuis, D.G. (1992). Aging, perceptual and cognitive functioning and interactive
equipment. In: H. Bouma & J.A.M. Graafmans. (Eds.). Gerontechnology. (pp. 93-112).
IOS Press, Amsterdam. ISBN 90-5199-072-3.

Brekel, H. van den. (1998). Oud van dagen. Vergrijzing in Nederland, 1970-1997.
Demos, 14(2), http://www.nidi.nl/public/demos/dm98024.html

Brandtstädter, J. & Renner, G. (1990). Tenacious goal pursuit and flexible goal
adjustment: Explication and age-related analysis of assimilation and accommodation
strategies of coping. Psychology and Aging, 5, 58-67.

Brink, S. (Ed.). (1998). Housing older people: an international perspective.
Transaction Publishers, London. ISBN 0-7658-0416-6.

Campbell, P., Dries, J. & Gilligan, R. (1999). The older generation and the European
information society: access to the information society. Final project report:
Recommendations for policy makers, NGO's and industry.
European Institute for the Media, Duesseldorf. ISBN 90-76299-04-8.

Charness, N. (Ed.). (1985). Aging and human performance: Studies in human
performance. Wiley, New York. ISBN 0-471-90068-0.

Charpentier, F. & Moulines, E. (1998). Pitch-synchronous waveform processing
techniques for text-to-speech synthesis using diphones. Eurospeech, 2, 13-19.

Collis, C. & Mallier, T. (1998). Government and the provision of training for older
workers. In: J. Graafmans, V. Taipale & N. Charness. (Eds.). Gerontechnology:
A sustainable investment in the future. (pp. 381-384).
IOS Press, Amsterdam. ISBN 90-5199-367-6.

Craik, F.I.M. & Bosman, E.A. (1992). Age-related changes in memory and learning.
In: H. Bouma & J.A.M. Graafmans. (Eds.). Gerontechnology. (pp. 79-92).
IOS Press, Amsterdam. ISBN 90-5199-072-3.

Craik, F.I.M. & Salthouse, T.A. (2000). The Handbook of aging and cognition, 2nd Edition. Lawrence Erlbaum Associates, Publishers, Hillsdale, N.J.
ISBN 0-8058-2966-0.

Czaja, S. & Glascock, A. (Eds.). (1994). Technology and environmental issues for the elderly. Experimental Aging Research, 20(3, Special issue).
Taylor and Francis, Washington D.C. ISSN 0361-073X.

Docampo Rama, M. & Kaaden, F. van der. (in press). Technology generations: characterisation on the basis of user interface changes.
Proceedings of the 3rd International Congress on Gerontechnology, Munich.

Doets, C. & Huisman, T. (1997). Digital skills. The state of art in the Netherlands.
CINOP, 's Hertogenbosch.

Durinck, J.R. (1996). The study of health and aging in relation to work.
In: W.J.A. Goedhard. (Ed.). Aging and Work 3, (pp. 37-47).
ICOH Scientific Committee Aging and Work, [S.l.]. ISBN 90-803145-1-X.

Duvanto, S., Huuhtanen, P., Nygard, C.H. & Ilmarinen, J. (1995).
Performance efficiency and its changes among aging municipal workers.
Scand J Work Environ Health, 17 (suppl. 1), 118-121.

Electronic House Magazine. Enhanced lifestyles through home electronics.
EH Publishing, Inc., Wayland. ISSN 0886-6643.

Elias, J.W. (Ed.). (1994). Aging and driving. Experimental aging research, 20(1, Special issue). Taylor and Francis, Washington D.C. ISSN 0361-073X.

Emerit, I. & Chance, B. (Eds.). (1992). Free radicals and aging.
Birkhauser Verlag, Basel. ISBN 0-8176-27448.

Eurolink Age. (1994). Mobility and transport, Meeting the needs of older people with disabilities. Report from a Eurolink Age seminar, Brussels, November 5-7, 1993.
Eurolink Age, London.

European Commission (1996). European Commission Green Paper. The citizens' network: Fulfilling the potential of public passenger transport in Europe. COM(95), 601final. http://europa.eu.int/en/record/green/gp9601/ind_cit.htm

Fernie, G.R. (1992). A modular support system to aid safer mobility.
In: H. Bouma & J.A.M. Graafmans. (Eds.). Gerontechnology. (pp. 223-228).
IOS Press, Amsterdam. ISBN 90-5199-072-3.

Fisk, A.D. & Rogers, W.A. (Eds.). (1996). Handbook of human factors and the older adult. Academic Press, San Diego. ISBN 0-12-257680-2.

Fozard, J.L. & Heikkinen, E. (1998). Maintaining movement ability in older age: challenges for gerontechnology. In: J. Graafmans, V. Taipale & N. Charness. (Eds.). Gerontechnology: A sustainable investment in the future. (pp. 48-60).
IOS Press, Amsterdam. ISBN 90-5199-367-6.

Fozard, J.L. (2000). Sensory and cognitive changes with age. In: K.W. Schaie & M. Pietrucha. (Eds.). (2000). Mobility and transportation in the elderly. (pp. 1-44).
Springer Publishing, New York. ISBN 0-8261-1309-5.

Fozard, J.L., Rietsema, J., Bouma, H. & Graafmans, J.A.M. (2000, in press) Gerontechnology: Creating enabling environments for the challenge and opportunities of aging. Educational Gerontology.

Giniger, S., Dispenzieri, A. & Eisenberger, J. (1983). Age, experience and performance on speed and skill jobs in an applied setting.
Journal of Applied Psychology, 68, 469-475.

Glenn, N.D. (1977). Cohort analysis.
Sage Publications, Beverley Hills. ISBN 0-8039-0794-X.

Goedhard, W.J.A. (Ed.). (1992). Aging and work 1.
ICOH Scientific Committee Aging and Work, [S.l.]. ISBN 90-9005032-9.

Goedhard, W.J.A. (Ed.). (1996). Aging and work 3.
ICOH Scientific Committee Aging and Work, [S.l.]. ISBN 90-803145-1-X.

Goedhard, W.J.A. (Ed.). (2000). Aging and work 4: healthy and productive aging of older employees. [s.n., S.l.]. ISBN 90-803145-3-6.

Golant, S.M. (1992). Housing America's elderly.
Sage publications, Newbury Park, CA. ISBN 0-8039-4763-X.

Goor, A.G. van de & Becker, H.A. (2000). Technology generations in the Netherlands: a social analysis. Shaker, Maastricht.

Graafmans, J.A.M. & Brouwers, A. (1989). Gerontechnology, the modeling of normal aging. In: Proceedings of the 33rd annual meeting of the Human Factors Society, Denver, Colorado, October 1989. (pp. 187-190).
The Human Factors Society, Santa Monica, CA. ISSN 0163-5182.

Graafmans, J., Taipale, V. & Charness, N. (Eds.). (1998). Gerontechnology: A sustainable investment in the future. Proceedings of the second International Conference on Gerontechnology, Helsinki, October 1996.
IOS Press, Amsterdam. ISBN 90-5199-367-6.

Habraken, N.J. (1970). Three R's for housing.
Scheltema & Holkema, Amsterdam. ISBN 90-6060-014-2.

Halliwell, B. & Gutteridge, J.M.C. (Eds.). (1998). Free radicals in biology and medicine. 3rd Edition. Oxford University Press, Oxford. ISBN 0-19-850045-9.

Hämäläinen, H. & Vaarama, M. (1992). Evergreen, a microcomputer simulation in the planning of services for the elderly. In: H. Bouma & J.A.M. Graafmans. (Eds.). Gerontechnology. (pp. 431-433). IOS Press, Amsterdam. ISBN 90-5199-072-3.

Hannon, J.R., Bossone, C.A. & Wade, C.E. (1990). Normal physiological values for conscious pigs used in biomedical research. Laboratory Animal Science, 40(3).

Harrington, T., Graafmans, J., Hermens, Y. & Weerd, W. de. (1998). Shade tree psychophysics: Models, mathematical and concrete, for the simulation of ageing. In: J. Graafmans, V. Taipale & N. Charness. (Eds.). Gerontechnology: A sustainable investment in the future. (pp. 115-117). IOS Press, Amsterdam. ISBN 90-5199-367-6.

Ilmarinen, J. (Ed.). (1993). Aging and work 2. FIOH, Helsinki. ISBN 951-801-915-0.

Ilmarinen, J. & Tuomi, K. (1993). Workability index for aging workers. In: J. Ilmarinen. (Ed.). Aging and work 2. (pp. 142-151). FIOH, Helsinki. ISBN 951-801-915-0.

Ilmarinen, J. (1996). Productivity in late adulthood - physical and mental potentials after the age of 55 years. In: W.J.A. Goedhard. (Ed.). Aging and work 3, (pp. 3-16). ICOH Scientific Committee Aging and Work, [S.l.]. ISBN 90-803145-1-X.

Ilmarinen, J. & Louhevaara, V. (1996). FinnAge action programme: Respect for the ageing. In: W.J.A. Goedhard. (Ed.). Aging and work 3, (pp. 221-225).
ICOH Scientific Committee Aging and Work, [S.l.]. ISBN 90-803145-1-X.

Ilmarinen, J., Tuomi, K. & Klockars, M. (1997) Changes in the work ability of active employees over an 11-year period. Scand J Work Environ Health, 23 (suppl 1), 49-57.

Ioannou, P.A. (1997). Automated highway systems.
Plenum Press, New York. ISBN 0-306-45469-6.

Karwowski, W. (Ed.). (2000). International encyclopedia of ergonomics and human factors. Taylor and Francis, London. ISBN 0-7484-0847-9.

Kovar, M.G. & La Croix, A.Z. (1987). Aging in the eighties, ability to perform work-related activities. National Center for Health Statistics Advance Data, 136, 1-12.

Kuchinomachi, Y. et al. (1997). The relationship between the usability of daily electric appliances and the deterioration in cognitive function of old people. In: Proceedings of the 13th triennial Congress of the International Ergonomic Association. 5, 591-593.

Laflamme, L. & Menckel, E. (1995). Aging and occupational accidents: A review of the literature of the last three decades. Safety Science, 21, 145-161.

LaPlante, M.P., Hendershot, G. E. & Moss, A.J. (1997). The prevalence of need for assistive technology devices and home accessibility features.
Technology and Disability, 6(1-2), 17-28.

Lawton, M.P. (1989). Environmental proactivity and affect in older people.
In: S. Spacapan & S. Oskamp. (Eds.). The social psychology of aging.
Sage, Newbury Park (CA). ISBN 0-8039-3555-2.

Lawton, M.P. (1998) Future society and Technology. In: J. Graafmans, V. Taipale & N. Charness. (Eds.). Gerontechnology: A sustainable investment in the future.
(pp. 12-22). IOS Press, Amsterdam. ISBN 90-5199-367-6.

Leliveld, W.H. & Waterham, R.P. (1992). Using speech technology in the field of aids for the handicapped and elderly. In: H. Bouma & J.A.M. Graafmans. (Eds.).
Gerontechnology. (pp. 373-383). IOS Press, Amsterdam. ISBN 90-5199-072-3.

Levón, B-V. & Kaakinen, J. (1998). Safety for the elderly by improving the environment. In: J. Graafmans, V. Taipale & N. Charness. (Eds.). Gerontechnology: A sustainable investment in the future. (pp. 362-364). IOS Press, Amsterdam.
ISBN 90-5199-367-6.

Lewin, K. (1951). Field theory in social science: selected theoretical papers.
Harper and Row, New York.

Lopes Cardozo, R., Spruit, R. & Suyderhoud, F. (1977). Hofjes in Nederland.
Gottmer, Haarlem. ISBN 90-257-0935-4.

Lundervold, D. A. & Poppen, R. (1995). Biobehavioral rehabilitation for older adults with essential tremor. The Gerontologist, 35(4), 556-559.

Masthoff, J.F.M. (1997). An agent-based interactive instruction system. Ph.D. dissertation. Eindhoven University of Technology, Eindhoven. ISBN 90-386-0319-3.

McEvoy, G.M. & Cascio, W.F. (1989). Cumulative evidence of the relationship between employee age and job performance. J. of Applied Psychology, 74(1), 11-17.

Medina, J.J. (1996). The clock of ages: why we age, how we age, winding back the clock. Cambridge University Press, Cambridge. ISBN 0-521-46244-4.

Merk, H.F. & Jugert, F.K. (1993). Metabolic activation and detoxification of drugs and xenobiotica by the skin. In: R. Gurny & A. Teubner. (Eds.). Dermal and Transdermal Drug Delivery. (pp. 91-100). Wissenschaftliche Verlagsgesellschaft mbH, Stuttgart. ISBN 3-8047-1223-1.

Meydani, M. (1992). Vitamin E requirement in relation to dietary fish oil and oxidative stress in elderly. In: I. Emerit & B. Chance. (Eds.). Free radicals and aging. (pp. 411-418). Birkhauser Verlag, Basel. ISBN 0-8176-27448.

Moraal, J. (1993). Aging and work. In: K. Broekhuis, C. Weiers & J. Moraal. (Eds.). Aging and human factors. Proceedings of the Europe chapter of the Human Factors and Ergonomics Society. (pp. 7-18). University of Groningen, Groningen. ISBN 90-6807-311-7.

Mutsuhashi, T. (1998). Human-friendly broadcasting technology. NHK R&D 50, 53-59.

Noorden, L. van & McEwan, J. (1992). Pilot applications for advanced communication technology in care for the elderly in Europe. In: H. Bouma & J.A.M. Graafmans. (Eds.). Gerontechnology. (pp. 271-276). IOS Press, Amsterdam. ISBN 90-5199-072-3.

Norman, D.A. (1988). The psychology of everyday things. Basic Books, New York. ISBN 0-465-06709-3.

Norman, D.A. (1993). Things that make us smart: Defending human attributes in the age of the machine. Addison-Wesley, New York. ISBN 0-201-58129-9.

OSHA (Occupational Safety and Health Administration, US Department of Labor). Occupational Safety and Health Standards, Part 1910 Subpart Z. Toxic and hazardous substances. Hazard communication. - 1910.1200. http://www.osha.gov

Pauzié, A. & Letisserand, D. (1992). Ergonomics of mmi in aid driving systems: approach focusing on elderly visual capacities. In: H. Bouma & J.A.M. Graafmans. (Eds.). Gerontechnology. (pp. 329-334). IOS Press, Amsterdam. ISBN 90-5199-072-3.

Placencia Porrero, I. & Ballabio, E. (Eds.). (1998). Improving the quality of life for the European citizen. IOS Press, Amsterdam. ISBN 90-5199-406-0.

Ricklefs, R.E. & Finch, C.E. (1995). Aging: a natural history. Scientific American Library, Oxford. ISBN 0-7167-5056-2.

Rogers, W.A., Fisk, A.D. & Walker, N. (Eds.). (1996). Aging and skilled performance. Lawrence Erlbaum Associates, Publishers, Mahwah, N.J. ISBN 0-8058-1909-6.

Rowe, J.W. & Kahn, R.L. (1998). Successful aging.
Pantheon Books, New York. ISBN 0-375-40045-1.

Russell, L. (1999). Housing options for older people.
Age Concern, London. ISBN 0-8624-2287-6.

Salthouse, T.A. (1984). Effects of age and skill in typing.
Journal of Experimental Psychology, (113) 3, 345-371.

Saranummi, N. (1997). Ageing and technology: state of the art.
European Commission Joint Research Centre, Sevilla. EUR 17285 EN.

Schaie, K.W. & Pietrucha, M. (Eds.). (2000). Mobility and transportation in the elderly.
Springer Publishing, New York. ISBN 0-8261-1309-5.

Scharf, B. & Buus, S. (1986). Audition 1: Stimulus, physiology, thresholds.
In: K.R. Boff, L. Kaufman & J.P. Thomas. (Eds.). Handbook of perception and human performance, Volume 1. (pp. 14.1-14.71). Wiley-Interscience, Chichester.
ISBN 0-471-88544-4.

Schieber, F. (1992). Aging and the senses. In: J.E. Birren, R.B. Sloane & G.D. Cohen. (Eds.). Handbook of mental health and aging. Academic Press, San Diego.
ISBN 0-12-101277-8.

Schneider, E.L. & Row, J.W. (Eds.). (1996). Handbook of the biology of aging.
4th Edition. Academic Press, London. ISBN 0-12-627873-3.

Slangen-de Kort, Y. (1999). A tale of two adaptations. Coping processes of older persons in the domain of independent living. Ph.D. dissertation.
Eindhoven University of Technology, Eindhoven. ISBN 90-386-0799-7.

Snel, J. & Cremer, R. (Eds.). (1994). Work and aging: a European perspective.
Taylor & Francis, Hampshire. ISBN 0-7484-164-4.

Spirduso, W.W. (1995). Physical dimensions of aging.
Human Kinetics, Champaign, IL, USA. ISBN 0-87322-323-3.

Spirduso, W.W. (1995). Balance, posture and locomotion.
In: W.W. Spirduso. Physical dimensions of aging. (pp.155-184).
Human Kinetics, Champaign, IL, USA. ISBN 0-87322-323-3.

Statistics Netherlands/Statline, the statistical database on the Netherlands.
http://argon2.cbs.nl/statweb/indexned.stm

Steenbekkers, L.P.A. & Beijsterveldt, C.E.M. van (Eds.). (1998). Design-relevant characteristics of ageing users: Backgrounds and guidelines for product innovation. Delft University Press, Delft. ISBN 90-407-1709-5.

Stewart, T. (1992). Physical interfaces or "obviously it's for the elderly, it's grey, boring and dull." In: H. Bouma & J.A.M. Graafmans. (Eds.). Gerontechnology. (pp. 197-207). IOS Press, Amsterdam. ISBN 90-5199-072-3.

Tacken, M., Marcellini, F., Mollenkopf, H. & Ruoppila, I. (Eds.). (1999). Keeping the elderly mobile. Outdoor mobility of the elderly: problems and solutions. TRAIL Conference Proceedings Series No. P99/1. Delft University Press, Delft. ISBN 90-407-1930-6.

Tamura, T., Togawa, T., Ogawa, M. & Yamakoshi, K. (1998). Fully automated health monitoring at home. In: J. Graafmans, V. Taipale & N. Charness. (Eds.). Gerontechnology: A sustainable investment in the future. (pp. 280-284). IOS Press, Amsterdam. ISBN 90-5199-367-6.

Traffic Safety Facts (1994). US Department of Transportation. National Center for Statistics and Analysis, Washington D.C.

Transportation Research Board (1998). Transportation in an aging society. TRB, special report 218. TRB, Washington D.C.

Tsang, P.F. & Shaner, T.L. (1998). Age, attention, expertise and time-sharing performance. Psychology and Aging, 13, 323-347.

Verhelst, W.D.E. (1991). A system for prosodic transplantation with research applications. IPO Annual Progress Report, 26, 29-38.

Welford, A.T. (1951). Skill and age: An experimental approach. Published for the Nuffield Foundation by the Oxford University Press, London.

Welford, A.T. (1958). Ageing and human skill. Published for the Nuffield Foundation by the Oxford University Press, London.

WHO Study Group on Aging and Working Capacity. (1993). Aging and working capacity. WHO technical report series no. 835. World Health Organization, Geneva. ISBN 92-4-120835-X.

Woollacott, M.H. & Shumway-Cook, A. (Eds.). (1989). Development of posture and gait across the life span. University of South Carolina, Columbia. ISBN 0-87249-629-5.

World Health Organization. (1998). The World Health Report. Life in the 21st century: a vision for all. World Health Organization, Geneva. ISBN 92-4-156189-0.

Yu, Byung Pal. (1993). Free radicals in aging. CRC Press, London. ISBN 0-8493-4518-9.

Keyword index

A

AARP 131, 132, 149
accessibility 68, 69, 79, 126
accident 32, 67, 70, 78, 120, 132
    prone 51, 90
ADA 125
adjustable 61, 82, 91, 154
age 7, 8, 10, 18, 22, 28, 31, 55, 77, 162, 188, 189
    simulation 20, 26, 79, 117, 165, 167, 169, 170, 179
agent architecture 146
aging 2, 7, 10, 12, 13, 30, 34, 37, 42, 48, 54, 74, 166, 168, 171, 179
    biological aging............................ 111
airplane 107, 115, 123, 128
Alzheimer, see dementia
ambitions 2, 4, 14, 24, 192, 196, 203
ambulation 77, 169
animal model 54, 55, 96
antioxidant 49, 52
architecture 146
assistive devices 102
assistive technology 34, 156, 192
attitude 35, 63, 88, 128, 189
automatic features 61
average fallacy 61

B

balance 33, 60, 69, 77, 78, 116
bathroom 68, 70, 78
bear's favor 17, 30
bus 12, 33, 123, 126
bus system, see homebus

C

cane 25, 33
car 34, 115, 116, 123
care 3, 25, 27, 109, 135
    care assist 159
chemical awareness 71
chronic diseases 38, 87
cognition 204
communal facilities 62
communication 135, 139, 145, 155
compensation 3, 25, 102, 103, 105, 125, 130, 133, 153, 196
control 4, 15, 77, 80, 142, 152
control systems 177
controls 72, 104, 163, 203
Cost A5 .... 35, 193
cultural differences 63, 64
customization 74, 103, 150

D

DAN 194
data collection 183
decline 28, 77, 86, 89, 121
dementia 22, 60, 116
demography 10
design 15, 17, 33, 78, 149, 151
    for all 153
diabetes 44, 46, 47
diet 7, 48, 49,
digestion 37
disability 25, 61, 117, 125
diversity 16
domotics 72, 75 79
driving 34, 118, 128, 132, 133

217

E

education 35, 100, 101, 126
e-mail 21, 24, 188
endurance 32
enhancement 3, 24, 108, 133, 156
environment ... 1, 24, 39, 41, 68, 73, 126, 179
    living 197, 202, 203
    technological 4, 148, 187
    working 97, 104, 151
ergonomics 35, 61, 88
ETAN-expert group 194
ethical 119
Eurolink Age 36, 126, 194
European Commission 5, 38, 76, 123, 194
exercise 24, 37, 52, 199

F

falls 78, 97, 118, 169
fear of technology 15, 187
fertility rate 10
fitness 25, 39
flexibility 17, 72, 104, 112, 150
foresight 175
free radicals 42, 46, 49, 52, 56

G

gait 169
gender 8, 16, 51, 54
gerontechnology 2, 4, 7, 12, 13, 20, 24, 34, 39, 53, 60, 187
    definition 2, 35
    history 34
    International Society for 5, 198
gerontology 2, 7, 30
glucose monitoring 44
group painting 157

H

handicap 33, 87, 155, 192
hazards 33, 39, 69, 78, 96, 119
health . 1, 27, 37, 39, 49, 51, 82, 88, 203
    health promotion 88, 105
    health education 199

health technology 197
hearing 31, 99, 144, 151, 154, 162
    hearing aid 162, 193
    hearing threshold 31, 151, 154
help function 15
hofjes 62
home bus 72, 76
house mites 73, 202
housing 59, 60, 63, 64, 74, 179

I

ICT 15, 24, 139, 190, 193
immobility 115
impairments 38, 192
independence 1, 8, 63, 192
individual differences 14, 28, 91
information ergonomics 190, 192
instruction 143
insulin 44, 46, 47
intelligent transport system 129, 130
interface 80, 146, 151, 158
Internet 46, 139, 149, 188

J

JRC-study 194

K

Kaizen 95

L

learning 15, 142, 143, 191, 193
    situated learning 193
    lifelong learning 110
life expectancy 10, 37, 38, 51
life style 40, 49, 82, 111, 165
locomotion 33, 75, 137

M

medical surveillance 109
memory 191
    prospective memory 191
    working memory 89, 191
metabolic 47
metabolism 50
mites, see house mites

mobility 115, 122, 133, 135
   outdoor mobility 115
model 165, 174, 178
   deterministic model...................... 174
   game theory.................................. 175
   mathematical model 26, 27, 137, 165, 174, 181, 183
   predictive model 174, 175
   stochastic model........................... 174
model house 79
modeling 118, 165, 178
monitoring.. 25, 40, 44, 46, 52, 178, 202
moving 77, 115

N

networks... 139
nutrition................................. 37, 50, 51

O

oxidative stress............................. 42, 43

P

PDA 153
performance monitor....................... 199
personal... 79
   personal digital assistant 153
   personal housing 59
   personal mobility 115, 135, 136
physical ability 74
physical exercise 52, 98
plane, see airplane
pollutants..................................... 71, 73
prediction 168, 175
prevention 2, 24, 25, 40, 50, 51, 78, 82, 94, 98, 99, 120, 122, 145, 148, 149, 151, 203
privacy 66
protection 71, 75, 99
psychophysics 21, 32, 136, 171
public health................................... 7, 41
Public Health Engineering . 41, 197, 202
public transportation 115, 119, 123
pulmonary functioning...................... 73

Q

quality of life 4, 192, 203

R

RD&D 2, 25, 35
reaction time 22, 108, 124, 132, 171
regulation..96
remapping..155
research 3, 24, 25, 54, 111, 136, 161
retirement 65, 85, 92, 93, 108

S

safety 32, 40, 67, 78, 96, 121, 131
scenario 175
security 79, 80
Senior label................................68, 74
simulation 20, 26, 165, 167, 169, 179
situated learning 193
smart house................................79, 80
speech 144, 151, 162
stigmatizing 92

T

taxi..123, 126
telework...104
telomeres 48
toilet..................................68, 81, 82
toxicity..55, 96
train 99, 115, 123
training 98, 101, 106, 110, 111, 122, 128, 143, 148
transport system...............................126
transportation..........................115, 128
traveling...115
tremor 20, 106, 170

U

useful field of view...........................121
user interface ..4, 15, 104, 146, 155, 190
   adaptive interface 192
   generic user interface 193, 203

V

validity 183
vibration 31
vision 21, 22, 32, 79, 122, 161, 172, 191
visual field 79, 151, 169
vulnerability 37, 43, 97, 202

W

walking 74, 115, 116, 128
way finding 75
wheelchair 68, 128
WHO 85, 86, 88, 89, 111
work ability index 87
working 85, 111
   working environment 87, 112
   working capacity 88
WWW 18, 55, 72, 161

Author index

AARP, 131
Aberson, 191
Anan, 204
Ausman, 54
Bailer, 29
Ball, 121
Ballabio, 192
Baltes, M.M., 196
Baltes, P.B., 196
Becker, 189
Beijsterveldt, 60, 83
Bezooijen, 99
Birren, 36, 56
Blaich, 80
Bosman, 191
Bossone, 54
Bouma, 15, 34, 36, 61, 164, 191, 192, 204
Bouwhuis, 164, 191
Brandtstädter, 196
Brekel, 19
Brink, 83
Brouwers, 34
Buus, 31
Campbell, 204
Cascio, 102
Chance, 56
Charness, 36, 112, 204
Charpentier, 144
Collis, 101
Craik, 191, 204
Cremer, 112
Czaja, 204
Dispenzieri, 90
Docampo Rama, 189
Doets, 140
Dries, 204
Durinck, 109
Duvanto, 108

Eisenberger, 90
Elias, 137
Emerit, 56
Eurolink Age, 36, 126, 194
European Commission, 123
Fernie, 30
Finch, 56
Fisk, 36, 204
Fozard, 60, 116, 137, 204
Gilligan, 204
Giniger, 90
Glascock, 204
Glenn, 189
Goedhard, 110, 112
Golant, 83
Goor, 189
Graafmans, 34, 36, 179, 185, 204
Graves, 206
Gutteridge, 56
Habraken, 83
Halliwell, 56
Hämäläinen, 27
Hannon, 54
Harrington, 169, 179, 185
Heikkinen, 60
Herbig, 82
Hendershot, 211
Hermens, 179, 185
Huisman, 140
Huuhtanen, 208
Ilmarinen, 85, 87, 92, 93, 98, 112, 208
Ioannou, 129
Jugert, 97
Kaaden, 189
Kaakinen, 78
Kahn, 205
Karwowski, 204
Klockars, 210
Kovar, 74, 98

Kuchinomachi, 155
La Croix, 74, 98
Laflamme, 98, 105
LaPlante, 60
Lawton, 15, 188, 196
Legein, 191
Leliveld, 155
Letisserand, 161
Levón, 78
Lewin, 196
Lopes Cardozo, 62
Louhevaara, 93
Lundervold, 106
Mallier, 101
Marcellini, 137
Masthoff, 164, 193
McEvoy, 102
McEwan, 147
Medina, 48, 56
Mélotte, 191
Menckel, 98, 105
Merk, 97
Meydani, 52
Mollenkopf, 137
Moraal, 23
Moss, 211
Mosteller, 29
Moulines, 144
Mutsuhashi, 144
Noorden, 147
Norman, 164
Nygard, 208
Ogawa, 82
OSHA, 55, 57, 113
Owsley, 121
Pauzié, 161
Pietrucha, 137
Placencia Porrero, 192
Poppen, 106
Renner, 196
Ricklefs, 56
Rietsema, 204

Rogers, 36, 204
Row, 56
Rowe, 205
Ruoppila, 137
Russell, L., 83
Russell, R.M., 54
Salthouse, 22, 23, 204
Saranummi, 195, 205
Schaie, 36, 137
Scharf, 31
Schieber, 130, 185
Schneider, 56
Shaner, 130, 185
Shumway-Cook, 60
Slangen-de Kort, 196
Snel, 112
Spirduso, 36, 46, 60, 118, 137
Spruit, 62
Steenbekkers, 60, 83
Stewart, 15, 164
Suyderhoud, 62
Tacken, 137
Taipale, 36
Tamura, 82
Thomas, 206
Togawa, 82
TRB, 137
Tsang, 130, 185
Tuomi, 87
Vaarama, 27
Vercruyssen, 128
Verhelst, 144
Wade, 54
Walker, 204
Waterham, 155
Weerd, 179, 185
Welford, 22, 23
WHO, 11, 85, 86, 105, 112, 205
Woollacott, 60
Yamakoshi, 82
Yu, 56
Zabel, 191

Table of boxes

Box 1.1 Demography of age	10
Box 1.2 Technophobia?	15
Box 1.3 Change in sex ratio	18
Box 1.4 Choice reaction time versus typing	22
Box 1.5 Misinterpretation of experimental results	28
Box 2.1 Public Health Engineering	41
Box 2.2 Management of diabetes	44
Box 2.3 Telomeres: The fuses of aging?	48
Box 2.4 Gender differences in health	51
Box 2.5 Research misses the aging	54
Box 2.6 Research on toxicity	55
Box 3.1 Cultural differences in housing	64
Box 3.2 Senior label for housing	68
Box 3.3 Domotics	72
Box 3.4 Home bus standardization	76
Box 3.5 Domestic hazards	78
Box 3.6 Smart toilet	82
Box 4.1 Work ability index	87
Box 4.2 Japan's "Kaizen" way to help older workers	95
Box 4.3 Training for older workers	101
Box 4.4 Voluntary work	110
Box 5.1 Citizen's network	123
Box 5.2 Technology and the bicycle	127
Box 5.3 Smart roads	129
Box 6.1 Use of ICT by older people	140
Box 6.2 Slowed listening	144
Box 6.3 Videophone	147
Box 6.4 Senior net	149
Box 6.5 Warning signals	154
Box 6.6 Signal-to-noise ratio of speech	162
Box 7.1 Advantages of modeling	168
Box 7.2 Four layer model	176
Box 7.3 Simulation of aging in the house	179
Box 8.1 Technology generations	189

Box 8.2 Networking with other scientific organizations 191
Box 8.3 Some programs in Europe 194
Box 8.4 International Society for Gerontechnology (ISG) 198
Box 8.5 Gerontechnology research across the world 200

Table of figures

Percentage of people living independently in the Netherlands	8
Life expectancy at birth in various continents	10
Decrease in total fertility rate over the years worldwide	11
Ratios of females to males in the United States in different age groups	18
Predicted ratios of females to males in the United States in various age groups	19
Choice reaction time and typing speed as a function of age	22
Data of an unpublished experiment on word remembering as a function of age	28
Thresholds for hearing as a function of age	31
Overview of regions for the promotion of health	39
Mean distance (in km) traveled by bicycle per day in 1996 in the Netherlands	127
Self-test on speed of reaction	132
Usage of information related equipment as a function of age in the Netherlands	140
Schematic sound spectra of beeper and mechanical bell as compared to average hearing thresholds of young and old subjects	154
Letter size wedge	172